Communication Skills for Medicine

Third Edition

Professor Margaret Lloyd MD FRCP FRCGP
Emeritus Professor of Primary Care and Medical Education,
University College Medical School, University College London

Professor Robert Bor MA (Clin Psych) DPhil CPsychol CSci FBPsS FRAeS
UKCP Reg EuroPsy
Consultant Clinical Psychologist, Royal Free Hospital, London

Contributions by

Geraldine Blache MSc CPsychol
Chartered Psychologist and Organisational Consultant, London

Zack Eleftheriadou MA MSc CPsychol & Chartered Scientist UKCP Reg
Dip Infant Mental Health
Psychologist and Integrative and Psychoanalytic Psychotherapist, Visiting Lecturer
Tavistock Clinic and private practice, London

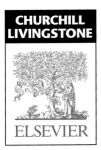

CHURCHILL
LIVINGSTONE

ELSEVIER

EDINBURGH LONDON NEW YORK OXFORD PHILADELPHIA ST LOUIS SYDNEY TORONTO 2009

CHURCHILL
LIVINGSTONE
ELSEVIER

© 2009, Elsevier Limited. All rights reserved.

First edition 1996
Second edition 2004
Third edition 2009

ISBN 978-0-7020-3058-1

British Library Cataloguing in Publication Data
A catalogue record for this book is available from the British Library

Library of Congress Cataloging in Publication Data
A catalog record for this book is available from the Library of Congress

Notice
Neither the publisher nor the authors assume any responsibility for any loss or injury and/or damage to persons or property arising out of or related to any use of the material contained in this book. It is the responsibility of the treating practitioner, relying on independent expertise and knowledge of the patient, to determine the best treatment and method of application for the patient.

The Publisher

ELSEVIER
your source for books, journals and multimedia in the health sciences
www.elsevierhealth.com

Working together to grow
libraries in developing countries

www.elsevier.com | www.bookaid.org | www.sabre.org

ELSEVIER   BOOK AID International   Sabre Foundation

The Publisher's policy is to use **paper manufactured from sustainable forests**

Printed in China

Preface

The first edition of this book was published in 1996 and since then communication skills teaching has continued to develop in both undergraduate and postgraduate education. The intended outcome is to educate a generation of doctors who can communicate effectively and sensitively with patients, relatives and colleagues.

Many doctors increasingly recognise that communication skills in medical practice are not simply about positive engagement with patients. Effective communication also helps us to understand better a patient's problem, the impact it has on the patient's life and relationships and also how best to manage the problem in the patient's life. Nowadays, effective communication skills are also vital for reducing the risk of error in clinical practice as well as avoiding complaints about one's practice. Both of these could have serious consequences for the doctor. There is no formula or short-cut for learning communication skills as we have to engage differently with each patient. There are, however, certain approaches and skills that help us to communicate more effectively, and the evidence strongly suggests that communication skills can be taught and learned. Since the last edition there has been more research in all aspects of communication in medicine and we have tried to reflect this in the text and references.

The principles that gave guidance in our writing of the first edition have not changed. We set out to produce a practical guide to the learning and development of communication skills that would be of value to students throughout their careers. The order of the chapters reflects this development from basic communication skills to those required in dealing with challenging situations. We have maintained the same format as the first edition, including case examples, guidelines and opportunities to encourage the reader to 'stop and think'. The skills of effective, sensitive communication are learnt and developed by practising them and reflecting on the process. We hope that the exercises and the appendices will help students and their teachers to do this.

All of the chapters have been revised and references updated. A new section on medical professionalism has been added in response to the increasing emphasis now placed on professionalism and the role of the doctor in society.

We hope that this book will continue to provide students and teachers with a map to guide their learning and teaching of the skills of good communication.

M.L.   London
R.B.   2008

Foreword

The ten years or more since the first edition of this fine book was published have been one of the most exciting periods in the development of the medical sciences. The completion of the human genome project, surely one of the most remarkable achievements in human biology, was followed by predictions that medicine would change completely over the next 20 years and that many of our intractable diseases would be preventable or at least amenable to improved forms of therapy. As the dust has settled on this heady period, however, it has gradually become clear that human beings are even more complex organisms than was ever imagined. And although some progress has been made in applying our new technology to the prevention and control of disease it is now clear that we have only the flimsiest ideas about the workings of healthy bacteria, never mind the multi-layered and infinite complexity of sick people.

In my small monograph, *Science and the Quiet Art*, I pointed out that while we should make every effort to explain our patients' problems in the language of modern science, in many cases, because of ignorance a moment would come when we would have to call on the classical skills of good doctoring, including sympathetic communication skills, an ability to carry out a painstaking clinical examination, but above all to be able to listen to what our patients have to tell us. However far modern science is able to move medical care forward, these skills, particularly an ability to listen and develop an attitude of humility, will always be required for good medical practice.

As witnessed by the new edition of this book, it is possible to do a great deal to improve doctors' communication skills and, along the way, improve their facility for listening to what their patients are telling them. Paradoxically, the extraordinary advances in the basic medical sciences, which are pointing daily to our profound ignorance about what makes us what we are, may engender a greater humility in our profession, so vital for generating skills in communication and listening.

None of the richer countries of the world has learnt how to cope with the increasing costs and pressures of medical care, particularly those that result from their increasing aged populations. The pressure on doctors, whatever their field, are enormous and it is increasingly difficult for them to spend adequate time talking to their patients. But as this book clearly states, there are no short cuts to medical communication skills, a message that has to be stated absolutely clearly to those who control and organise our health services. Modern medical technology can never be used as an excuse for a five minute consultation. Sadly, these are issues which our governments continue to fail to understand.

Clearly, there is still an enormous need for a book of this kind. The appearance of its third edition is a clear witness to its value and I wish it all the success it deserves in the future.

D.J. Weatherall
November 2008

Contents

1. Introduction   *1*
2. Basic communication skills   *9*
3. The medical interview   *28*
4. Giving information   *49*
5. Breaking bad news   *60*
6. Taking a sexual history   *77*
7. Communicating with patients from different cultural backgrounds   *89*
8. Guidelines on communicating with children and young people   *111*
9. Communication with a patient's family   *126*
10. Mistakes, complaints and litigation   *139*
11. Challenging consultations: special problems in doctor–patient communication   *147*
12. Communicating with patients and colleagues: learning more about how personal issues affect professional relationships   *170*

Exercises   *187*
Appendix A: Guidelines for using role-plays   *195*
Appendix B: Guidelines for giving feedback   *197*
Appendix C: Assessment of communication skills   *198*
Appendix D: Presentation: hints and assessment   *203*
Further reading   *205*
Subject Index   *207*

1

Introduction

> "Communication is not an 'add-on' – it is at the heart of patient care."[1]

> "Good communication is difficult: few can master it without special tuition and constant attention to its effectiveness."[2]

The aim of this book is to help you to develop the skills that will enable you to communicate effectively and sensitively with patients and their relatives and with your colleagues. The importance of good communication between patients and those who care for them cannot be disputed. However, as we shall see later, patients' experiences of the care they receive often fall far short of the ideal. With the exciting technological advances being made in clinical medicine, it is easy to be swept along by the science of medicine and to forget the ancient aim of the physician: 'To cure sometimes, relieve often, comfort always'.

The ability to communicate well with patients – to build up a trusting relationship within which curing, relieving and comforting can take place – is a great challenge that, as Sir Charles Fletcher pointed out,[2] should always be before us. Thirty years later, the General Medical Council in the UK has reinforced this in their latest recommendations on undergraduate education:[3]

> "Graduates must be able to communicate clearly, sensitively and effectively with patients and their relatives, and also colleagues from a variety of health and social care professions."

What is communication?

STOP AND THINK

This may seem a question with an obvious answer. But is it? What does the word 'communication' mean to you? Do some brainstorming, either by yourself or in a group. Write down all the words or phrases which come to mind. Think about:

- *a definition of communication*
- *the methods of communication*
- *the purpose of communication.*

Some things you may have thought of are shown in Figures 1.1 and 1.2.

1

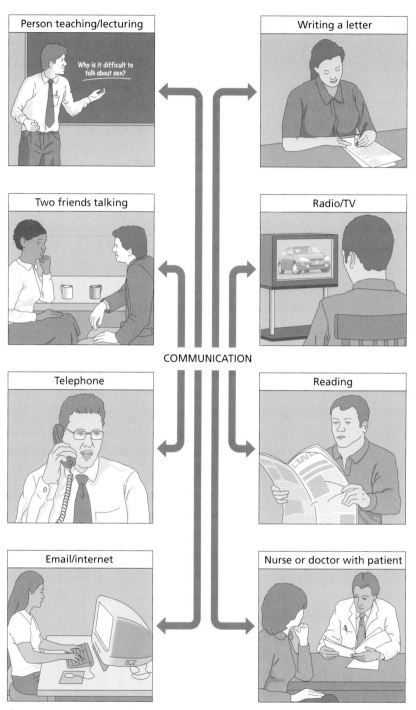

Fig. 1.1 Some methods of communicating.

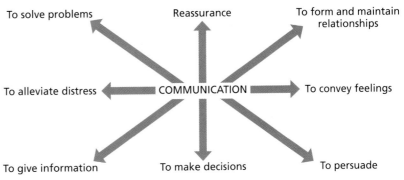

Fig. 1.2 Some purposes of communicating.

The *Oxford English Dictionary* tells us that the word 'communicate' comes from the Latin 'to impart, to share'. 'Communication' is imparting, conveying or exchanging ideas and knowledge.

What is good communication?

We shall deal with this in detail in the next chapter, but it is appropriate here to mention a study carried out some years ago by Dr Peter Maguire and colleagues in Manchester.[4] Patients who had been interviewed by medical students were asked for their opinion of the students' interviewing abilities. Patients preferred interviewers who:

- were warm and sympathetic
- were easy to talk to
- introduced themselves
- appeared self-confident
- listened to the patients and responded to their verbal cues
- asked questions that were easily understood and were precise
- did not repeat themselves.

Why is good communication important?

The short answer is 'better care for our patients'. There is considerable evidence to show that doctors who communicate well with patients are more likely to:

1. make an accurate, comprehensive diagnosis. Good communication skills enable one to collect information about a patient's problems that is comprehensive, relevant and accurate. It has been shown that doctors who have received training in communication skills are more likely to diagnose psychiatric morbidity in their patients than those who have not been trained.
2. detect emotional distress in patients and respond appropriately.
3. have patients who are satisfied with the care they have received and who are less anxious about their problems.
4. have patients who agree with and follow the advice given.

There is also evidence that good communication can have a positive effect on the patient's physical condition. One study showed that patients with hypertension who had been allowed to express their concerns about their problem had a significantly greater reduction in their blood pressure than those who had not been given this opportunity but had been treated similarly in other respects.[5] A study carried out in general practice showed that patients presenting with sore throat were more likely to get better sooner if they felt they were able to discuss their concerns with the doctor.[6]

Unfortunately, it is not difficult to find examples of the consequences of poor doctor–patient communication. A study in Florida[7] compared patients' opinions of obstetricians who had had malpractice claims made against them with those who had not been sued. It was found that patients were most likely to complain about aspects of patient–doctor communication rather than the technical aspects of care. The most frequent complaints about the doctors were that they:

- would not listen
- would not give information
- showed lack of concern or lack of respect for the patient.

The link between poor communication and complaints by patients will be discussed further in Chapter 10. In countries where patients are less likely to sue their doctors, patients also express dissatisfaction about how doctors communicate and relate to them. A report of a survey carried out in the UK includes a quote from a patient with breast cancer:

"They just told me I was going to have a mastectomy. No choice, no explanation. They don't discuss much with patients. I would have preferred that they had explained more.[1]*"*

This survey was reported in 1993 and, although there is now greater emphasis on providing patients with information and explanation, it is important to remember that most complaints are still related to a breakdown in communication.

Can communication skills be learned?

Training to be a doctor involves the acquisition of knowledge, skills and appropriate attitudes. Like many aspects of medical education, it was assumed until fairly recently that students acquire good communication skills and appropriate attitudes by a sort of osmosis – by observing and modelling their behaviour on that of their teachers.

As we have already seen, however, this may not produce doctors who are good communicators. It is now recognised that the apprenticeship method is not sufficient and that formal training in communication skills is necessary and effective. Medical schools have responded by introducing communication skills as a formal and important part of the curriculum and assessments.

What is the evidence for the effectiveness of communication skills training?

In the 1970s a series of studies was carried out on medical students during their fourth-year clerkship in psychiatry.[4] The study found that, before training, students experienced difficulties in obtaining histories from patients. The difficulties which were highlighted included:

- not obtaining all the necessary information from the patient
- forgetting to ask about the influence of the patient's problems on him- or herself and family
- failing to notice and respond to verbal and non-verbal cues from the patient
- looking bored during the interview.

As part of these studies a group of students were divided into a control group and a feedback group. In order to assess their baseline interviewing skills, students in both groups were asked to interview a patient and obtain a history of the patient's main problems within 15 minutes. The interviews were videotaped and the students were asked to write up the patient's history. The feedback group then interviewed two more patients and were also videotaped. However, on these occasions the students watched and discussed their interviews with a tutor during a feedback session, comparing it with an instructional handout. Finally both the control group (who had had no training) and the feedback group made a final videotaped interview with a patient. These interviews and the pre-training interviews were then rated and given a score by a psychologist who was blind to whether a student had received training or was a control.

What were the results?

It was found that the students who had received feedback training were better at communicating with patients because:

- compared to the control group, they obtained three times more relevant and accurate information about the patient's presenting problem
- they were given higher ratings by the patients.

Similar studies have been carried out by other workers, and most have demonstrated that students who receive training are better at communicating with patients than untrained students.

Another question must be asked. Are the skills that these students acquired through training retained, or are they lost over a period of time? Further studies using the same experimental design were carried out on both groups 4–6 years later.[4] The studies showed that the doctors who had received video feedback training as students retained their skills:

- They were more empathic.
- They were more self-assured when interviewing patients.

- They had better basic communication skills, including the use of an open style of questioning and responding to verbal cues.

Further studies have produced strong evidence that communication skills can be learned and retained.[8,9]

How to develop good communication skills

The most important point to realise is that you have the ability to communicate and that you use this ability continually when relating to other people. Learning communication skills is, therefore, different from learning, for example, to take someone's blood pressure, which you are unlikely to have done before coming to medical school. The communication skills courses that are now part of the curriculum in all medical schools aim to help you to hone your innate skills and develop specific skills that enable you to communicate effectively with patients. Communication skills training will enable you to identify these skills and practise them with your fellow students or simulated patients (often actors role-playing patients). This is important for learning how to take a history from a patient, but even more important for situations when communication may be particularly difficult for both you and the patient, for example when you have to tell a patient that he or she has cancer, or when you need to take a sexual history.

These situations are never easy to cope with, but it does help if you have been able to practise the necessary skills and explore your own feelings about these issues with other students and a tutor in a supportive setting.

So, what is the best way to learn the skills of effective communication? Clearly, this will depend on your teachers' experiences and opinions. However, there is evidence from Maguire's work that students learn communication skills most effectively if the following conditions are fulfilled:

- Students are given written instructions about the information to be obtained from training and the skills to be used.
- The skills are demonstrated by the teacher.
- Students are given opportunities to practise these skills with real or simulated patients under controlled conditions.
- Students are given feedback on their performance by audio- or video-taped replay.
- Students are able to discuss their performance and related issues with a tutor.

Finally, here is a cautionary note. You may think that you have excellent communication skills and will have no problems in dealing with patients. You may be tempted to say: 'Communication skills seminars are not for me – I don't need them'. However, one study of medical students has shown that students who are the most confident tend to be least competent in communicating with patients.

Lifelong learning

Remember that learning to communicate well does not stop at the end of the undergraduate course. We all need to develop and hone our communication skills with patients, relatives and colleagues throughout our professional lives. This is now recognised in the postgraduate examinations, where communication skills are now formally assessed.

How to use this book

We hope the book will help you to develop your communication skills. It takes a practical approach and concentrates on the patient–doctor/ student relationship. Where appropriate, it discusses both oral communication with colleagues and written modes of communication. Throughout, you will find the following features that we hope will aid your learning.

'Stop and think' boxes

These aim to encourage you to pause in your reading, to marshal your thoughts and to reflect on your own experiences. There is considerable evidence that we learn best if we can link new knowledge and skills to what we already know and can do, and if we make use of and practise what we have acquired. In other words, learning must be an active process.

Exercises

These should be used as part of active learning. They are grouped together towards the end of the book. Each exercise refers to a section in the book, where reference is made to it.

Guidelines

These are 'how to do it' summaries intended to be helpful. They are meant to guide you and should not be treated as directions.

Key points

The important messages contained in each chapter are summarised at the end of the chapter.

Case examples

These are an important part of the book and are intended to make the clinical situations come alive for you.

Appendices

These are concerned with the process of teaching communication skills and should be particularly useful to those involved in teaching students.

FURTHER READING

Silverman J, Kurtz S, Draper J 2005 Skills for communicating with patients, 2nd edn. Radcliffe Medical Publishing, Oxford

REFERENCES

1. Audit Commission 1993 'What seems to be the matter?': communication between hospitals and patients. HMSO, London
2. Fletcher CM 1973 Communication in medicine. Rock Carling monograph. Nuffield Provincial Hospital Trust, London
3. General Medical Council 2002 Tomorrow's doctors: recommendations on undergraduate medical education. HMSO, London
4. Maguire P, Fairbairn S, Fletcher C 1989 Consultation skills of young doctors: benefits of undergraduate feedback training in interviewing. In: Stewart M, Roter D (eds) Communicating with medical patients. Sage Publications, California
5. Kaplan SH, Greenfield S, Ware JE 1989 Assessing the effects of physician–patient interactions on the outcomes of chronic disease. Medical Care 27: S110–S127
6. Little P, Willamson I, Warner G et al 1997 Open randomised trial of prescribing strategies in managing sore throat. British Medical Journal 314: 722–727
7. Hickson GB, Clayton EW, Entman SS 1994 Obstetricians' prior malpractice experience and patients' satisfaction with care. Journal of the American Medical Association 272: 1583–1587
8. Aspergren K 1999 Teaching and learning communication skills in medicine: a review with quality grading of articles. Medical Teacher 21: 563–570
9. Yedida MJ, Gillespie CC, Kachur E et al 2003 Effect of communication skills training on medical student performance. Journal of the American Medical Association 290: 1157–1165

2

Basic communication skills

In Chapter 1 we saw the importance of communicating effectively and sensitively with patients, and that these skills can be learned. In this chapter we are going to examine these skills in more detail. But first we need to look briefly at the factors that influence communication and, in particular, doctor–patient communication.

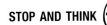 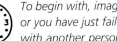

To begin with, imagine that you have some bad news (e.g. a relative has just died, or you have just failed some exams) and that you decide to share this information with another person. Think about the factors that:

- *would help you to begin to share the information*
- *would hinder you sharing information.*

First of all, the setting or situation is clearly important – you are unlikely to discuss how you feel if the conversation takes place on the top of a bus or in a crowded room. Secondly, how you feel at the time will influence what you say, and so will the attitude of the other person – both at the start of the conversation and during it. You are more likely to be able to share information and to find the process helpful if the other person is friendly and attentive. Similarly, the sharing of information between patient and doctor can be influenced by factors that relate to the setting of the interview and to each of the participants.

Patient-related factors influencing communication

People cope with illness in different ways depending upon their personality, upbringing, social class, ethnic and cultural background and their life experiences. These factors will influence how they communicate (Table 2.1). Reactions to illness include denial, anger, anxiety and depression. These responses will determine if and when a person seeks medical attention and will also influence a patient's behaviour when receiving care.

Most people experience a degree of anxiety and apprehension when consulting a doctor. In particular, admission to hospital is a disturbing

Table 2.1 Factors which influence doctor–patient communication
Patient-related factors <ul><li>Physical symptoms</li><li>Psychological factors related to illness and/or medical care (e.g. anxiety, depression, anger, denial)</li><li>Previous experience of medical care</li><li>Current experience of medical care</li></ul> **Doctor-related factors** <ul><li>Training in communication skills</li><li>Self-confidence in ability to communicate</li><li>Personality</li><li>Physical factors (e.g. tiredness)</li><li>Psychological factors (e.g. anxiety)</li></ul> **The interview setting: requirements** <ul><li>Privacy</li><li>Comfortable surroundings</li><li>An appropriate seating arrangement</li></ul>

experience for most of us. Factors that contribute to our anxiety include an unfamiliar environment, loss of personal space, separation from family and friends, loss of independence and privacy and uncertainty about diagnosis and management. Thus, individuals' physical condition and their psychological state related to both their illness and the medical care they receive will influence the communication process. As we shall see later, it is important to identify and seek to overcome patient-related factors (e.g. anxiety) that may impair communication.

Other factors that must be taken into account are:

- the patient's beliefs about health and illness
- the problem the patient wishes to discuss
- the patient's expectations of what the doctor will do (often based on previous experience)
- how the patient perceives the role of the doctor.

Doctor-related factors

Some medical students and doctors find it easier than others to empathise and communicate with patients, although, as we have already noted, these attributes can be acquired by training. Other factors influence our behaviour during a consultation (Table 2.1). As a medical student you may initially find it difficult when interviewing patients who are much older than yourself, particularly when sensitive issues such as sexual behaviour are involved. It is not difficult to understand why a medical student just before finals, a junior doctor at the end of a long shift or a GP who has already seen two dozen patients earlier in the morning may have less to give a particular patient. Tiredness, anxiety and preoccupation with other concerns are all likely to impair communication, and we need to be aware of these limitations. We also need to be aware of our own prejudices and take care that they do not interfere with our communication with patients. For example, a patient who persistently presents with symptoms that do not appear to have a physical basis must be taken seriously, and must not be dismissed as a hypochondriac. These issues are discussed in greater detail in Chapter 12.

The setting of the interview

Most consultations take place in a hospital ward, the outpatient clinic or the GP's surgery. In each case every effort should be made to provide a setting that facilitates communication (Table 2.1). Privacy is essential. A patient in a hospital bed is unlikely to divulge personal, sensitive information if she knows that Mrs Smith in the bed next door can hear every word through the curtains. If you do not feel that the setting is right, try to find an alternative (the majority of wards have interviewing rooms which ensure privacy), providing, of course, that the patient can be moved. Try to avoid interruptions and make sure that the lighting and temperature are as comfortable as possible. It is important to consider the arrangement of seats; they can influence how people communicate with each other and may give clues to how they perceive their own and each other's roles in the encounter. In the outpatient clinic or GP's consulting room, where there are usually chairs and a desk or a table, there are three possible ways of arranging the seating (Fig. 2.1).

Arrangement (a), with the patient and doctor facing each other across a desk, is unlikely to make the patient feel at ease or facilitate discussion, although the doctor may feel in control of the interview. Arrangements (b) and (c) are more informal and more likely to facilitate good communication.

Another point to consider is the distance between the interviewer and the patient. Placing seats too close together may make the patient feel threatened, while too far apart may convey a feeling that the interviewer is not interested in what the patient is saying. Most consultations take place at a distance of 1.25–2.75 metres (4–9 feet), although the distance may change during the course of the interview, e.g. as the doctor, you might draw your chair closer to the patient when offering reassurance.

Interviewing a patient who is in a hospital bed deserves special consideration. Standing over a patient is likely to increase the patient's feeling of vulnerability and should be avoided. It should always be possible to draw up a chair so that you are on the same level as the patient.

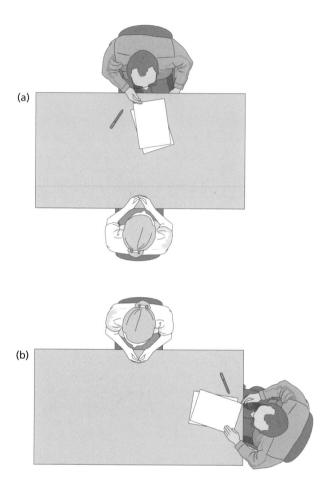

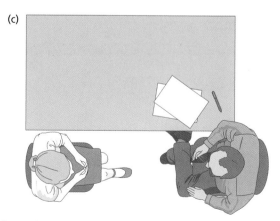

Fig. 2.1 Alternative seating arrangements in an interview.

Beginning an interview

The setting and the way in which we begin a conversation can have a profound effect on what follows. The aim in a formal setting should be to make the interviewee feel at ease. How can this be done?

STOP AND THINK

Think back to a formal interview in your own experience:

- *How did you feel before and during the interview?*
- *Did anything help to put you at ease? If so, what?*
- *Did anything make you feel uneasy? If so, what?*
- *What could have been changed to make you feel more comfortable?*

In describing what made you feel at ease, you might have included:

- a comfortable setting
- being greeted by name and a handshake
- being shown where to sit
- the interviewers introducing themselves and explaining the procedure
- an easy first question
- the interviewer appearing interested in your remarks.

Unfortunately, interviewers may neglect some or all of these strategies, and doctors are no exception. An unsatisfactory beginning is likely to lead to an unsatisfactory consultation, as the following case illustrates.

Case example 2.1

How not to begin an interview

Mrs Francis, a shop assistant aged 31, attended medical outpatients at her local hospital. Here is her story:

"When I went into the room, which was big and bare, I felt lost. I didn't know where to sit, the doctor had his head down and was writing, the nurse was on the telephone and there were some medical students talking to each other. I waited around and wanted to run out the door. After what seemed like ages the doctor told me to sit down and asked what was wrong. I didn't know his name and I'm not sure that he knew mine. I'd been thinking about my problems and what I wanted to tell the doctor – but I forgot it all – he didn't seem very interested anyway. Hope I don't have to go again."

It is not difficult to spot what was wrong with the way this interview was conducted. By following simple rules, you can help patients feel at ease, and you can begin to build up a relationship that enables your patients to share the story of their illness with you. Beginning the interview involves greeting the patient, introducing yourself and orienting the patient (Table 2.2).

Much of the doctor's behaviour is simply common sense and courtesy, but this may be easy to forget or ignore, particularly when time is short.

Table 2.2 Guidelines for conducting an interview

Beginning the interview
- Greet the patient by name ('Good morning, Mr Richardson') and shake hands, if it seems appropriate
- Ask the patient to sit down
- Introduce yourself ('I am Judy Williams, a medical student')
- Explain the purpose of the interview ('I would like to find out about your present problem')
- Say how much time is available
- Explain the need to take notes and ask if this is acceptable

The main part of the interview
- Maintain a positive atmosphere, warm manner and good eye contact
- Use open questions at the beginning
- Listen carefully
- Be alert and responsive to verbal and non-verbal cues
- Facilitate the patient both verbally ('Tell me more') and non-verbally (using posture and head nods)
- Use specific (closed) questions when appropriate
- Clarify what the patient has told you
- Encourage the patient to be relevant

Ending the interview
- Summarise what the patient has told you and ask if your summary is accurate
- Ask if the patient would like to add anything
- Thank the patient

The main part of the interview

Look back to page 9 and remember what you thought would help you to begin to share your news with the other person. Now think what that person could do to help you to continue to share your entire story. You probably would expect your friend to:

- ask appropriate questions
- listen attentively and demonstrate interest
- help you to continue if you get stuck.

Questioning, listening and facilitating are three of the key skills that enable us to communicate effectively with others (Table 2.2).

Asking questions

One of the purposes of interviewing a patient is to obtain information about the condition for which the patient is seeking help. The information must be accurate, complete and as relevant as possible. The most obvious and direct way to obtain information is to ask questions. However, studies of medical students and doctors have found that they often:

- ask too many questions and do not allow patients to tell their story in their own words
- ask questions that are too long, too complicated and confusing
- ask questions in such a way that they may bias the answers given
- ignore questions that patients may ask.

So it must be concluded that asking questions is a valuable skill that needs to be learnt.

Open and closed questions

Asking open questions enables you to obtain a great deal of information and also allows patients to tell their own story. Open questions should be used as much as possible, particularly at the start of the interview, e.g. 'Would you please tell me how you have been feeling in the past few days?' Asking specific (i.e. closed) questions gives patients little choice in the way they answer and usually elicits a 'yes' or 'no' answer, e.g. 'Have you been feeling unwell today?'

Case example 2.2

A patient's response to open and closed questions

Mr Clark is an accountant aged 47 years. He comes to the accident and emergency department following an attack of chest pain. He is seen first by Dr Yates:

Dr Yates: *I see from your notes that you have had some chest pain. Do you still have the pain?*

Mr Clark: *No, not now.*

Dr Yates: *Was it tight or dull?*

Mr Clark: *It seemed a very dull pain.*

Dr Yates: *Did it go down your arm?*

Mr Clark: *No, I don't think so.*

Dr Yates: *Did it get worse when you exercised?*

Mr Clark: *No, it didn't.*

Later, Mr Clark is seen by Dr Vale:

Dr Vale: *I understand that you have had pain. Would you please tell me more about it?*

Mr Clark: *Well, it was in my chest and it came on when I was sitting at my desk. It was a funny dull pain that stayed in the middle of my chest. I've had it a few times recently, always when I'm at work.*

Dr Vale: *Can you tell me what brings it on?*

Mr Clark: *Well, I was thinking about that. I've been very busy at work recently, and it seems to come on when I'm rushing to finish accounts. It also seems to happen when I feel worried about something.*

This example illustrates the advantages of using open questions and the disadvantages of closed questions: Dr Vale obtained considerably more information by using open questions than Dr Yates, who used closed questions.

An open style of questioning is preferable because:

● more relevant information can be obtained in a given time
● patients feel more involved in the interview
● patients can express all the concerns and anxieties about their problems; these may be missed if closed questions are asked.

However, using open questions does have some disadvantages:

● the interview may take longer and be more difficult to control
● some of the information may not be relevant
● recording answers may be more difficult.

The interview between Dr Yates and Mr Clark illustrates the limitations of a closed style of questioning:

● the information obtained is restricted to the questions asked
● the interview is controlled by the interviewer, who decides the content of the questions
● the interviewee has little opportunity to express concerns and feelings. This may make the patient feel frustrated.

However, closed questions are useful when it is necessary to obtain specific information that the patient has not given or when the patient is shy or withdrawn and does not readily provide information. Closed questions may also be appropriate when it is necessary to obtain a limited amount of factual information in a limited period of time, e.g. when a patient in casualty presents with a painful arm after a fall, you will need to know quickly the site of the pain and if movement is possible.

(p. 187)   **Exercise 1**   Do Exercise 1 to demonstrate the advantages and disadvantages of Open and Closed Questions.

Probing questions

It is usually necessary during the interview to use probing questions that help a patient to think more clearly about an answer he or she has given. Probing questions may be used to:

● clarify: What do you mean by that?
● justify: What makes you think that?
● check accuracy: You definitely took three tablets a day?

Questions to be avoided

The questions asked during an interview should be easily understood and asked in a way that does not influence the patient's response. Complex questions and leading questions should be avoided.

Complex questions that encompass several questions in one are likely to confuse both the patient and the interviewer. For example, how would you respond to the question, 'Did your vomiting start yesterday or today and have you had diarrhoea?' The chances are that only one part of the question would be answered.

Leading questions encourage the person responding to give the answer that the interviewer expects or wants. In the context of interviewing patients, leading questions may be useful as an opening ploy, but on the whole they are to be avoided for reasons that will become obvious. There are three types of leading question:

1. *Conversational*: can be used to open or stimulate conversation; they can encourage rapport, e.g. 'Aren't we having awful weather this year?'
2. *Simple*: these influence the patient to agree with the interviewer's viewpoint and should not be used, e.g. 'You don't sleep well, do you?'
3. *Subtle*: these use the wording of the question to influence the respondent. They should be avoided, but it is easy to use them without realising it.

A good example of how the wording of a question can influence the answer was shown in a study of the frequency of headaches in a group of individuals. When respondents were asked, 'Do you get headaches frequently and, if so, how often?' the average response was 2.2 headaches per week. When the question was slightly changed to, 'Do you get headaches occasionally and, if so, how often?' the average response was 0.7 headaches per week.

How should the question have been phrased to avoid subtly influencing the response?

Listening

In the setting of the medical interview, patients appreciate and respond positively to the doctor who listens carefully. Many studies have shown this. Listening is one of the most obvious components of the communication process, yet active or effective listening is one of the most difficult skills to acquire. The first step is receiving the message from the other person.

(p. 187) **Exercise 2** You may wish to try the group Exercise 2, Passing on the message. The group task involved listening to a message containing a lot of information. You probably found that information was lost as the message was passed on because there was so much to remember. Some judgement is required to ensure that the most important information is retained. The message was probably transmitted inaccurately as each person unwittingly changed it to what they heard and understood. When listening, we tend to rationalise information to fit in with our own experience.

What would help us to listen in such a way that information is registered and passed on accurately? Possible ways include:

● taking notes
● asking the speaker to repeat or clarify parts that are not clear
● checking that the information received is accurate by repeating or summarising it.

Listening involves not only receiving information, but also, and more importantly, being 'in tune' with the speaker and responding appropriately. This is *active* or *effective listening*. It is not easy, and demands effort and concentration. When interviewing a patient it is important to demonstrate that you are paying attention and trying to understand what the person is saying and feeling. The key features of active listening are:

● gathering and retaining the information accurately
● understanding the implications for the patient of what is being said
● responding to verbal and non-verbal signals or cues
● demonstrating that you are paying attention and trying to understand.

Picking up cues

Patients may be unable or unwilling to articulate their real concerns and feelings. However, they are likely to reveal something of these during the course of the interview, and it is important that their verbal and non-verbal cues are picked up.

Verbal cues

Listen carefully to the way patients describe their problems for signs of their underlying concerns. They may reveal these only if you respond appropriately to their verbal cues.

Case example 2.3

Picking up verbal cues

DR STONE: *Hello, Mrs Fine, come and sit down. How can I help today?*
MRS FINE: *I thought I'd come to see you, doctor, about my headaches.*
DR STONE: *Perhaps you could tell me more about these headaches.*
MRS FINE: *Well, they're really bad, and getting worse. They started soon after my mother died and now they're making me feel dizzy. I'm really worried about them.*
DR STONE: *Could you tell me why you are worried about them?*

Dr Stone has picked up one of the verbal cues. The other cue is that Mrs Fine relates the symptoms to her mother's death, and Dr Stone should go on to explore her reaction, e.g. 'Could you tell me more about how you felt after your mother's death?'

Non-verbal cues

We reveal a lot of information about ourselves and our feelings in our body language – the way we dress, our posture, gestures and facial expressions. When you interview a patient, you can learn a good deal by watching the patient enter the room (appearance, posture and gait). It is also important to be sensitive to the patient's body language during the interview.

Here are some examples of non-verbal cues:

- *Eye contact*: difficulty in maintaining eye contact may indicate that the patient feels depressed, embarrassed about what is being discussed or uninterested in the conversation. Conversely, excessive eye contact may indicate anger and aggression.
- *Posture*: the confident person will sit upright; the patient who feels depressed may sit slouched with head bent forward.
- *Gestures*: for example, an angry patient may sit with clenched fists whereas an anxious patient may wring the hands or tap the feet continuously.
- *Facial expressions*: sadness, anger and happiness.
- *The way the voice is used*: tone, timing, emphasis on certain words and vocalisation other than with words (this is sometimes called paralinguistics).

Demonstrating active listening

It is essential to show the patient that you are listening carefully. This can be done by appropriate use of eye contact, posture (e.g. sitting slightly forward facing the patient), nodding your head and saying 'hmm – go on'. You can also demonstrate active listening by asking questions directly related to or following on from the patient's last statement.

(p. 189) **Exercises 3 & 4**   Exercises 3 and 4 illustrate the importance of verbal and non-verbal listening skills.

Facilitation

This is an essential part of effective listening; the aim is to help patients to talk as fully as possible about their problems. You can help them verbally or non-verbally. Examples of verbal facilitation are:

"Please go on and tell me more about your pain."

"Yes, I understand — please continue."

Remember to give the patient time to respond after you have spoken. Non-verbal means of facilitation include adopting an appropriate posture, e.g. lean slightly forward towards the patient, maintain eye contact and nod your head at appropriate times.

Clarification

It is sometimes necessary to ask patients to clarify something they have said. This can be done in several ways:

"Please tell me exactly when your abdominal pain started."

"Can you describe the pain in more detail?"

"What do you mean by 'dizziness'?"

Reflection

Reflecting back to patients what they have just said may help them to proceed with their story, particularly when they may be finding it difficult to go on because of their feelings.

Helping the patient to be relevant

It is important to use your time as efficiently as possible. This may involve helping the patient not to stray from the main point of the interview. To do this, you should interrupt at an appropriate point and try to redirect the interview. For example:

"What you've just told me about your job is interesting, but I'd like to hear more about the headaches you've been having."

"It would help me to know more about the circumstances that bring on your chest pain."

Silence

Silent periods may make us feel uncomfortable, and there can be a temptation to rush in with another question. Try not to do this. Silences are valuable, giving the patient time to reflect on what has been said. Use them yourself to observe the patient, to reflect on the interview so far and to plan the next stage.

Signposting

Signposts on a road direct us towards our destination and keep us on the right track. In the same way, signposting during a consultation indicates to the patient what you want to discuss next and is a valuable part of effective communication. Examples of signposting are:

"And now I would like to ask you a few more questions about ..."

and:

"Thank you for discussing your problems with me and now I would like to examine you."

Signposting is helpful throughout the consultation and at the end when you summarise what has been said.

Summarising

At the end of a consultation summarise what the patient has told you, e.g. 'I'd like to make sure that I've understood you correctly. You told me that ...'. Summarising serves several important functions:

- It allows you to check the accuracy of the patient's story by providing the patient with an opportunity to correct any misunderstandings.
- It enables you to review the patient's story and deduce what else needs to be explored, and it allows you to 'buy time' if you get stuck and can't think of what to ask next.
- Summarising what has been said so far may help the patient to carry on discussing the problem – it is one method of facilitation.
- It may help you to keep the patient 'on track'.
- It can let the patient know that you have been listening carefully and are interested.
- It is an appropriate way to close an interview.

Ending an interview

It is important to leave sufficient time to end the interview properly (Table 2.2). The essential features you should remember are:

- Summarise what the patient has told you.
- Ask the patient to check the accuracy of what you have said.
- Ask the patient if you have left out any information that the patient feels is important.
- Enquire if the patient would like to add anything.
- End by thanking the patient, e.g. 'Thank you for talking to me; our time is now up'.

Touch

Touch is a powerful means of communication that we use to express a whole range of emotions, including tenderness, love and anger. Within the context of the doctor–patient relationship, touch can convey concern and empathy, and it can have a therapeutic effect in itself. However, touch must be used appropriately and with due regard to the sensitivities of the patient and to professional codes of conduct.

When should touch be used in the doctor–patient encounter? Clearly, there are no hard and fast rules. Shaking a patient's hand on meeting at the start of an interview is socially appropriate. Putting your arm around a distressed person to give comfort, or placing your hand on the arm of a patient who is having difficulty expressing thoughts and emotions conveys empathy, and this often helps the person to continue. Here are two general guidelines when touching patients:

● Try to assess the patient's likely response to being touched. You can pick up clues from the way in which the patient relates his or her story, the patient's posture and other aspects of body language.
● If you feel uncomfortable about touching patients, it is probably advisable not to do it – you might communicate your anxiety to the patient.

Communication during the physical examination

What we have discussed so far about touch applies to communication during the interview. Some different issues are concerned with touching during a physical examination. Remember that patients are likely to be very conscious of their vulnerability and the power of the doctor as they lie on the couch waiting to be examined. They may also feel embarrassed and anxious about what may be found. Try to put them at ease. Here are some guidelines:

● Always respect the patient's sensitivity and modesty; a blanket should be available to cover the patient before and during the examination.
● Explain what you are going to do. Does the patient have any concerns about this?
● Be careful not to instil anxiety at this stage by your facial expressions, or by spending a long time on one part of the examination without explanation.
● Avoid causing discomfort if possible by watching the patient's expressions or by saying, 'Please tell me if I am hurting you'.

Empathy

Patients appreciate the interviewer who demonstrates empathy. Empathy means putting yourself in the other person's place. As Sir William Osler advised: 'Realise as far as you can the mental state of the patient, enter into his feelings, scan gently his thoughts. The kindly word, the cheerful greeting, the sympathetic look – these the patient understands.'

Some people can empathise more easily than others by virtue of their personality. However there is evidence that the ability to empathise with a patient is a skill which can be learnt. Demonstrating empathy involves many of the skills we have discussed in this chapter, including:

- maintaining good eye contact with the patient and adopting an appropriate posture and tone of voice
- listening attentively
- picking up and responding to verbal and non-verbal cues from the patient
- indicating that you understand what is happening to the patient, e.g.:

> PATIENT: *My father died from a heart attack 7 years ago whilst I was on holiday in France.*
>
> DOCTOR: *That must have been a distressing time for you.*

Remember that empathy is a powerful therapeutic tool.

Patient-centred consultations

Traditionally doctors have taken the dominant role in a consultation, aiming to interpret the patient's symptoms from the perspective of disease and pathology. They have paid less attention to the patient's concerns and understanding of their illness, and have not involved the patient in decisions about their treatment. This has been called the doctor-centred style of communication and was accepted by most patients. However, this has changed and many patients want to know more about their illness and be involved in treatment decisions. Moreover, there is now increasing evidence that a more patient-centred style of consultation results in patients who are more satisfied, more likely to adhere to treatment and have better health outcomes.[1]

Many of the case examples in this book illustrate the patient-centred approach to interviewing patients. Here is an example which contrasts doctor-centred and patient-centred interviewing styles.

Case example 2.4

Doctor- and patient-centred interviewing styles

Mrs Fraser works as a clerk in an office. She has been referred to her local hospital by her GP because she has had a persistent cough and wheeze for the past 6 months. She has tried to stop smoking but is finding this difficult. Her cough is worse when she is at work and she is worried that it is brought on by the air conditioning in the office. She is afraid that she may have to leave her job, which she depends on to support herself and her three children.

Doctor-centred style

> DR ELIOT: *Your doctor says that you have a cough. How long have you had it for and is there anything else wrong?*
>
> MRS FRASER: *I've had it for 6 months and sometimes I wheeze.*
>
> DR ELIOT: *Do you smoke?*

MRS FRASER: *Well, I've been trying to stop and now I only smoke two cigarettes in the evening.*

DR ELIOT: *Your symptoms are probably due to your smoking. I strongly advise you to stop smoking. I'll arrange for you to have a chest X-ray and other tests and I'll see you in 1 month's time.*

Patient-centred style

DR ELIOT: *Your doctor says that you have a cough. Please could you tell me more about it and about any other symptoms you may have?*

MRS FRASER: *Well, I've had this cough for about 2 months now and sometimes I feel short of breath, particularly in the morning.*

DR ELIOT: *Could you tell me if you bring up any sputum when you cough?*

MRS FRASER: *Yes, sometimes I do in the morning but I think that's because I smoke, although I am trying to cut down. Also, I wheeze, particularly when I'm at work and I think that's due to the air conditioning.*

DR ELIOT: *You seem to have two concerns. First, you want to stop smoking and I am sure that this is important for your health. Second, you are worried about your work. How do you think that I can help?*

MRS FRASER: *Well, I would like some help to stop smoking and I wonder if you could write a letter to the doctor at work because I've had quite a lot of time off work recently. I'm really scared that I will lose my job and get behind with the mortgage.*

What are the features of a patient-centred interview?

The patient-centred approach to interviewing has been described as 'entering the patient's world to see illness through the patient's eyes'.

STOP AND THINK 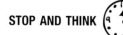 *How can you try to achieve this?*
First of all, look back at the two interviews between Dr Eliot and Mrs Fraser and list the differences between them.

The features of a patient-centred consultation are:

● Exploring the patient's experience of illness
● Exploring the patient's knowledge of his or her illness (communicating with the informed patient is discussed in Chapter 11)
● Allowing patients to express their beliefs about their illness, e.g. what caused it
● Allowing patients to express their concerns about the impact of their illness on their life
● Treating the patient as a partner when discussing treatment.

This is best achieved by practising the principles of good communication that we have outlined in this chapter:

- Helping the patient to feel at ease and adopting an empathic approach
- Using open questions
- Picking up and responding to verbal cues by listening actively to what the patient is saying
- Picking up and responding to non-verbal cues.

Is patient-centred interviewing always appropriate?

Apart from emergency situations, patient-centred interviewing is appropriate in most consultations and leads to better outcomes for the patient and doctor. However, it is important to remember that some patients prefer doctor-centred consultations, i.e. they want the doctor to take a more paternalistic approach and to take charge of the consultation and their treatment.

Professionalism and communication skills

You may have noticed when reading newspapers, magazines and medical journals that the term 'professionalism' is often mentioned and debated. Over the last few years the concept of professionalism has assumed increasing importance. Since the time of Hippocrates, medicine has been one of the most highly regarded of all the professions. This raises a number of questions, including: What is a profession? What does professionalism mean in the context of being a doctor?

  The professions include medicine, nursing and the law. What do these have in common? What are the characteristics of a profession?

A useful definition is that a profession has a body of specialist knowledge, is autonomous and is accountable to society. Its members are altruistic and trusted by members of society. Next, think about this in the context of being a doctor.

 What do we mean by 'medical professionalism'? Begin by thinking about the qualities and behaviour expected of a good doctor.

STOP AND THINK

You could begin by looking at the Hippocratic oath, which in the past was sworn by those entering the medical profession. Few, if any, medical schools require this now on graduation, although some schools hold white-coat ceremonies for incoming students who make promises reflecting some aspects of the oath.[2]

We may think that we know what professionalism is but then find it difficult to define. We can recognise professional behaviour and, perhaps more readily, when someone is acting unprofessionally. Many of the professional bodies have debated professionalism and have attempted to define it. Here is the definition from the Royal College of Physicians of London:

> *"Medical professionalism signifies a set of values, behaviours and relationships that underpins the trust the public have in doctors.[3]"*

These professional values, behaviours and relationships are expressed in the duties of a doctor, as listed by the UK's General Medical Council[4] (Table 2.3).

Table 2.3 The duties of a doctor[4]

- Make the care of your patient your first concern
- Protect and promote the health of patients and the public
- Provide a good standard of practice and care
- Treat patients as individuals and respect their dignity
- Work in partnership with patients
- Be honest and open and act with integrity

STOP AND THINK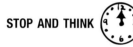

Think about the link between these duties and how you communicate with patients.

Some of these links have been discussed in previous chapters. Others have been identified by the General Medical Council in *Good Medical Practice* and are shown in *italics*:

- Make the care of your patient your first concern.
    - Look back at the sections on empathy, patient-centred consultations and professionalism.
- Protect and promote the health of patients and the public.
    - This involves giving lifestyle advice – see Chapter 4.
- Provide a good standard of practice and care.
    - This involves teamwork and maintaining your own skills.
- Treat patients as individuals and respect their dignity.
    - *Treat patients politely and considerately.*
    - *Respect patients' rights to confidentiality.*
- Work in partnership with patients.
    - *Listen to patients and respond to their concerns and preferences.*
    - *Give patients the information they want or need in a way they understand.*
    - *Respect patients' right to reach decisions with you about their treatment and care.*
- Be honest and open and act with integrity.

As you will see, developing and continuing to practise good communication skills is fundamental to fulfilling your duties as a doctor.

Key points

- Communicating effectively with patients involves the core skills of questioning, active listening and facilitating.
- These skills can be learned and need to be practised.
- Asking questions
  - Use open questions as often as possible, particularly at the beginning of an interview.
  - Obtain specific information using focused and closed questions.
  - Use probing questions to clarify, check accuracy and to help patients expand on what they have said.
  - Avoid using leading questions.
  - Avoid asking several questions at once: this is confusing.
  - Allow patients time to answer your question.
  - Rephrase a question using simpler language if they do not understand or if their answer is unclear.
- Listening
  - Listening is one of the core skills of good communication.
  - Allow patients to talk without interruption.
  - Effective listening means concentrating on what patients say and trying to understand their feelings as they speak.
  - Be alert to verbal and non-verbal cues.
  - To demonstrate your attention, use appropriate body language and facilitate comments.
  - Allow pauses or silences.
- Signposting
  - Use this throughout the consultation to introduce what you are going to say next.
- Leave time at the end of the interview to summarise what the patient has said and ask if the patient has anything to add.
- Some common pitfalls to be avoided are:
  - asking too many questions
  - not allowing patients to tell their story in their own words
  - unnecessary interruptions
  - failing to pick up important verbal and non-verbal cues.
- Professionalism
  - Good communication skills are an essential component of professional behaviour.

REFERENCES

1. Stewart MA, Brown JB, Weston WW et al 2003 Patient-centred medicine: transforming the clinical method, 2nd edn. Radcliffe Publishing, Oxford
2. Gillon R 2000 White coat ceremonies for new medical students. Journal of Medical Ethics 26: 83–84
3. Royal College of Physicians 2005 Doctors in society: medical professionalism in a changing world. Report of a working party of the Royal College of Physicians of London. Royal College of Physicians, London
4. General Medical Council 2006 Good medical practice. General Medical Council, London

3

The medical interview

"... the interview is potentially the most powerful, sensitive instrument at the command of the physician."

In these days of high-technology medicine this statement, made by George Engel in 1973, may surprise you. But the medical interview is still powerful and is likely to remain so. What is it that happens between doctor and patient that can make the interview such a powerful instrument?

Patients bring to the doctor their problems, usually in the form of symptoms or complaints, their anxieties about their problems and their concerns about other aspects of their life. They also have expectations about how the doctor will deal with them as a patient. The interview between patient and doctor is the cornerstone of the problem-solving process. The doctor's role is to gain as accurate a picture as possible of the patient's problems. This information must then be processed in such a way (usually in the form of making a diagnosis) that will enable the doctor, ideally in collaboration with the patient, to develop a plan for managing the problem. How is this done (Fig. 3.1)?

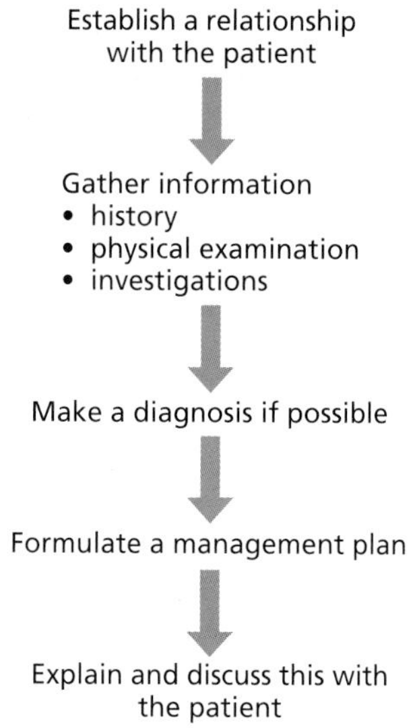

Establish a relationship with the patient

⬇

Gather information
• history
• physical examination
• investigations

⬇

Make a diagnosis if possible

⬇

Formulate a management plan

⬇

Explain and discuss this with the patient

Fig. 3.1 Developing a management plan for a patient.

1. Establish a rapport with the patient using the skills outlined in Chapter 2. This will enable the patient to tell his or her story, including underlying concerns, as completely as possible.
2. Use a framework for taking a medical history, as discussed later in this chapter.
3. Process the information acquired, supplemented by the results of the examination and appropriate investigations. This stage involves the knowledge of clinical medicine and decision-making processes that develop with experience. These will be discussed briefly later in this chapter.
4. Explain to the patient what may be wrong and how the patient might be helped. To do this successfully demands good communication skills and involving the patient in his or her management.
5. Close the interview by summarising what the patient has told you and thank the patient for his or her time.

Beginning an interview: establishing rapport

(p. 191) **Exercise 5** Review Chapter 2 and remember how important it is to provide a comfortable setting, to explain the purpose of the interview and to indicate the time available. Your aim is to help the patient to tell his or her story as fully and accurately as possible.

Case example 3.1

A good way to begin an interview

The senior registrar of a medical firm has asked one of the students to clerk Mr Jones, just admitted from casualty. The student finds that Mr Jones is in a side ward and is reading the newspaper when he enters the room.

STUDENT: *Hello, Mr Jones. I'm sorry to interrupt you but I'm Ben Brown, one of the students attached to Dr Morrison's firm. I've been asked to come and talk to you about the problem that brought you into hospital so that I can tell Dr Morrison about you when he does his ward round later this week. I can spend about 40 minutes talking with you. Is that all right?*

MR JONES: *Yes, sure – go ahead.*

STUDENT: *Well, I'd like to take some notes so that I can write up your history later. How do you feel about that?*

MR JONES: *That's fine by me.*

Gathering information: taking a medical history

A nineteenth-century French physician, René Laennec, advised: 'Listen to the patient. They are giving you the diagnosis'. His remark stresses the importance of a patient's history in making a diagnosis, and this has been confirmed in subsequent studies. One study found that in 66 of 80 patients, the correct diagnosis was made on the patient's history alone; in only 7 patients was the initial diagnosis changed after the physical examination; and in a further 7 it was changed after the results of investigations were available (Fig. 3.2).[1]

These findings underline the importance of gathering information from the patient as accurately and efficiently as possible using the skills outlined in Chapter 2. As suggested by Laennec, it is particularly important to listen attentively.

Often you will be asked to 'take a history from the patient' – an expression that implies that the process flows in one direction, from patient to doctor. But we have seen that what the doctor does (e.g. body language, manner of questioning and listening) influences how patients divulge their problems. It has been said that doctors should learn to receive, not to take, a medical history. Remember that you will obtain a more accurate and relevant history of the patient's problems if you develop good communication skills.

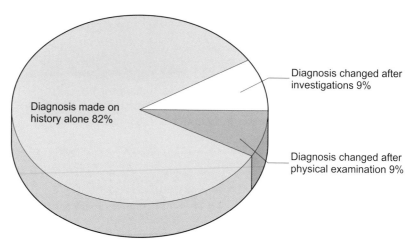

Fig. 3.2 Relative contribution of history, physical examination and investigations to final diagnosis.[1]

The structure of a medical history

When you begin your clinical training you will probably be given written instructions on 'how to take a medical history', and it is important to develop a system for taking a history based on this framework (Table 3.1).

Table 3.1 The structure of a medical history

- Basic information about the patient
- Description of presenting problem
- History of presenting problem
- Review of body systems
- Past medical history
- Family history
- Social history

Basic information about the patient

This includes the patient's name, address, age, occupation and marital status. You should try to find out the patient's name before the interview. If not, ask the patient his or her name and how he or she wishes to be addressed; the use of a person's Christian name is becoming increasingly common but many people, particularly older people, prefer the more formal mode of address. You may choose to gather the rest of the information during the course of the interview, which avoids beginning by asking the patient a list of questions.

Description of presenting problem

Find this out by asking an open question, e.g.:

"Could you please tell me what problem brought you to hospital?"

"Why have you come to see the doctor today?"

Record the patient's answer verbatim in the notes. Here are some examples from three patients:

MRS ALTON: *(a teacher, aged 52, married, with two children)*
My bowels haven't been right for some time now, and I've had this pain in my stomach.

MR BROWN: *(a retired garage owner, aged 72)*
I've had trouble passing my water.

MR DAWES: *(a builder, aged 47)*
I've had an attack of terrible pain in my chest, which is worrying me a lot.

Sometimes a patient will provide a diagnosis rather than a symptom: 'I have arthritis in my legs'. When this happens, it is important to ask the patient what he or she is experiencing: 'Could you tell me what symptoms you have?' The patient's understanding of arthritis might not be the same as yours. Don't be put off if the patient provides a diagnosis you have never heard of:

PATIENT: *Well, I have Osler–Rendu–Weber disease.*
STUDENT: *I'm afraid I don't know much about that disease yet – perhaps you could tell me how it troubles you.*

Patients may well not only describe their problems but also tell you about their condition: remember that patients can teach us a great deal.
A patient may describe his complaint in an emotional way:

MR DAWES: *I felt so awful that I thought I was going to die.*
DR BUCK: *That must have been very frightening. Do you want to talk about it now or shall we go on and talk about it later?*

It is important to acknowledge and respond to these emotions before continuing, even if it is decided to deal with the issues later on in the interview.
Next, ask the patient if he or she has any other problems. It is often easier to identify all the patient's problems before obtaining more information about the presenting complaint:

DR KITE: *You've told me that you have had trouble passing water. Before we discuss that further, could you tell me if you have any other problems?*
MR BROWN: *Yes, I've been a bit unsteady on my feet recently and a bit short of breath when climbing stairs, and I'm worried about my wife who has just had a stroke.*

Make a list of all the patient's problems – physical, psychological and social – to be dealt with in turn. This will help you to structure and pace the interview. It will also decrease the chance of the patient producing a problem (often the one that is worrying the patient most) just as he or she is about to leave the room. In this situation, you should never ignore the problem raised. The strategy you use to deal with it will depend on a number of factors, including the time available and how severe you think the problem is. You should give the patient an opportunity to describe the problem. If you feel it can be discussed at another time, you might say, 'Perhaps we can deal with that when you come to see me again tomorrow'.

Of course, patients may have problems that they have forgotten or may be reluctant to divulge at the start of the interview. But as you proceed and build up a rapport, patients may well feel able to discuss their problems with you.

History of presenting problem

This is one of the most important parts of the history (Fig. 3.3). Your aims should be to:

- obtain a detailed history that is complete, accurate and relevant
- find out the patient's perception of what is wrong
- establish the patient's attitudes to the problem
- determine what effect the problem has on the patient's day-to-day life and relationships.

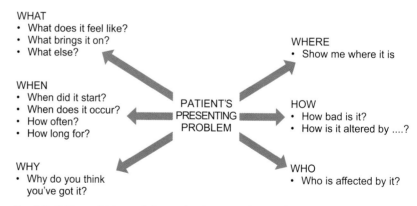

Fig. 3.3 Taking a history of the patient's presenting problem.

Now you can go on to gather a detailed history by asking further open questions. The exact nature of the questions will depend on the patient's problem. Most can be explored by asking:

WHAT: *What does it feel like? What brings it on?*
WHEN: *When did it start? When does it occur? (How often? How long for?)*
WHY: *Why do you think you have got it?*
WHERE: *Show me where it is.*

HOW: *How bad is it? How is it altered by food, exertion, etc.?*
WHO: *Who is affected by it?*

To look at this in more detail, we shall consider the questions that should be asked of a patient complaining of pain.

Timing: when?

You will need to know when the pain began, how it started, its duration, how often it occurs and, if appropriate, how it ended. Sometimes it is helpful to ask the patient to recall the onset of the problem and describe how it has developed since then. If there have been numerous different episodes, ask the patient to describe a typical one. It may be helpful to ask about the duration of pain:

DR BUCK: *How long does the pain last?*
MR DAWES: *Just a short while.*
DR BUCK: *A minute? Five minutes? Half an hour?*
MR DAWES: *Oh, not half an hour.*
DR BUCK: *How long then?*
MR DAWES: *About 15 minutes.*

Location: where?

This is particularly important when the patient complains of pain. It is a good idea to ask the patient to point to the site, e.g. if it is abdominal pain, you need to know the exact position in order to make the diagnosis.

Radiation: where?

It is also necessary to find out if the pain radiates and, if so, where the pain spreads to. A person with gallbladder disease may experience pain in the upper abdomen and in the right shoulder. Someone with a slipped disc may have back pain that spreads down the leg.

Quality: what is it like?

Symptoms vary in quality. For example, pain may be described as sharp, dull, tight, throbbing, constant or 'comes and goes'. The type of pain is important in differential diagnosis. For example, a patient with pleurisy will usually complain of chest pain that is sharp when breathing in, whereas someone who has had a heart attack will usually complain of constant 'tight, gripping pain' in the chest.

Severity: how bad is it?

You will want to know the severity of the problem, e.g. if pain is mild, moderate or severe. Of course, there is great variation in people's tolerance of pain, so it can be useful to ask patients to relate the severity of their present pain to a previous experience:

MR DAWES: *The pain was pretty awful.*
DR BUCK: *Would you say it is the worst pain you have ever had?*
MR DAWES: *Well, I had pain in my leg when I had sciatica, but this was far worse than that.*

Associated signs and symptoms: what else?

Asking about these can provide essential information for the diagnosis and management of the patient's condition:

DR BUCK: *When you had your chest pain, did you have any other symptoms at the time?*
MR DAWES: *Yes, my heart was racing and I felt a bit short of breath.*

This part of the history becomes easier as your knowledge of clinical medicine increases.

Setting: when does it occur?

It is important to establish the context in which the symptoms develop:

DR ROSS: *You have told me a lot about your abdominal pain and the way it's associated with wind and problems in passing your motions. Could you tell me now about what you are usually doing when the pain comes on.*
MRS ALTON: *I've been thinking about that. I never get this problem when I'm on holiday – it seems to happen mostly when I'm busy at work, or when we're expecting visitors at home.*

Modifying factors: how is it affected by . . . ?

Find out what makes the symptoms worse and what makes them better:

DR ROSS: *When you have the pain, is there anything that makes it better?*
MRS ALTON: *It's better when I've passed wind or had my bowels open.*
DR ROSS: *How does what you eat affect it?*
MRS ALTON: *I used to eat lots of vegetables and fruit, but I've cut that down and the pain seems to be a bit better.*
DR ROSS: *Do you ever take any medicines for the pain?*
MRS ALTON: *No. I tried paracetamol once, but that didn't seem to make any difference.*

The best way to obtain a history of the presenting complaint is to start with an open question, note which aspects of the problem the patient describes spontaneously, and then fill in the gaps with closed or probing questions. You may find this difficult to do initially, but it is a skill that comes with practice.

What effect does it have on the patient's quality of life?

You may have found out a lot about the impact of the problem on the patient's life from the patient's answers to your previous questions. You should look specifically at the effect on:

- mood
- relationships, particularly with spouse and close family
- job
- leisure and social life
- sexual activity.

> Dr Ross: *I'm wondering what effect your symptoms have had on your life in general.*
>
> Mrs Alton: *I'm not sure what you're getting at, but I know that they've made me feel a bit low at times.*
>
> Dr Ross: *A bit low? Can you explain what you mean by that?*
>
> Mrs Alton: *Well, I feel a bit fed up when the pain comes just before we're going out and I have to sit on the toilet for ages and then we're late – my husband gets really cross.*
>
> Dr Ross: *Does that worry you? Perhaps you could tell me how you are getting on with your husband?*
>
> Mrs Alton: *We've had our ups and downs – but not too bad, really.*
>
> Dr Ross: *And what about the rest of the family?*
>
> Mrs Alton: *Oh, my daughters are fine – we get on really well.*

Note how Dr Ross uses open questions, asks her to clarify what she means by 'a bit low', and picks up the verbal cues about her relationship with her husband.

What is the patient's understanding of the problem?

Try to explore what the problem means for the patient – what the patient thinks it might be caused by, or related to:

> *"Perhaps you could tell me what you think is causing your problem?"*

> *"What concerns you most about your problem?"*

It is important to get an understanding of patients' concerns and how they interpret their symptoms so that you can provide explanations and advice appropriate to their needs. This may be particularly important when a patient has a different cultural background to your own.

At this stage, try to summarise what the patient has told you about the present problem so that the patient can check the accuracy and fill in any gaps.

Review of body systems

This section of the interview involves a series of questions related to each of the body systems. The purpose is to elicit important symptoms that the patient may have forgotten or may not have considered significant because they were not related to their presenting complaint. Students often have a problem initially with this section of the interview: firstly, because of difficulty in remembering all the questions to be asked; and secondly, because they are afraid that the patient, who is likely to give negative answers to the majority of questions, may wonder about the questions' relevance. The way to overcome these problems is to:

● use an aide-mémoire: write down the body systems on a small card and refer to it in the interview
● introduce this section of the interview by saying something like: 'I'm now going to ask you a series of questions about common medical problems. This is to make sure we don't miss anything that may be important'.

The list of topics to be covered is shown in Figure 3.4. Examples of questions you might ask include the following.

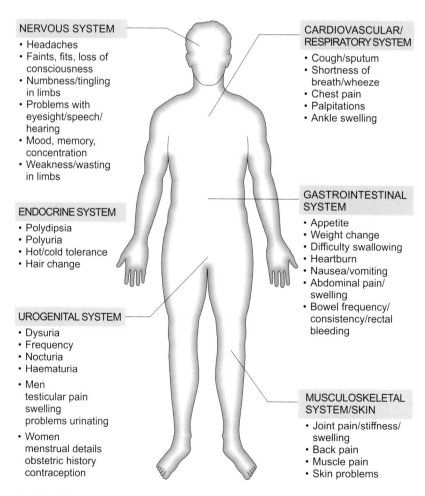

NERVOUS SYSTEM
• Headaches
• Faints, fits, loss of consciousness
• Numbness/tingling in limbs
• Problems with eyesight/speech/ hearing
• Mood, memory, concentration
• Weakness/wasting in limbs

ENDOCRINE SYSTEM
• Polydipsia
• Polyuria
• Hot/cold tolerance
• Hair change

UROGENITAL SYSTEM
• Dysuria
• Frequency
• Nocturia
• Haematuria
• Men
  testicular pain
  swelling
  problems urinating
• Women
  menstrual details
  obstetric history
  contraception

CARDIOVASCULAR/ RESPIRATORY SYSTEM
• Cough/sputum
• Shortness of breath/wheeze
• Chest pain
• Palpitations
• Ankle swelling

GASTROINTESTINAL SYSTEM
• Appetite
• Weight change
• Difficulty swallowing
• Heartburn
• Nausea/vomiting
• Abdominal pain/ swelling
• Bowel frequency/ consistency/rectal bleeding

MUSCULOSKELETAL SYSTEM/SKIN
• Joint pain/stiffness/ swelling
• Back pain
• Muscle pain
• Skin problems

Fig. 3.4 Systems review.

Cardiovascular

Could you tell me if you have any trouble with your heart? What about chest pain or palpitations? Do your ankles ever swell?

Respiratory

Do you have any problem with your lungs, like shortness of breath or coughing? Is sputum present? What colour it is? Have you ever seen blood in it?

Genitourinary

Do you ever have any problems passing water? What about pain when you pass it? Does your urine have an unusual colour or smell?

Assessment of the patient's mental state

This should form part of the interview with every patient. By carrying out a brief assessment of a patient's mental state, you can identify cognitive problems (which may alert you to the unreliability of the history) and the possibility of a psychiatric disorder. A brief account suitable for routine use will be given here. More detailed descriptions of assessment that should be followed if a psychiatric disorder is suspected are given in textbooks of psychiatry.

Appearance and behaviour

Non-verbal cues are particularly important in the assessment of a patient's mental state. Take particular notice of dress and general appearance. Patients who are demented or who are alcohol-dependent often neglect their appearance; the depressed patient may arrive dressed in sombre colours. During the interview, take note of the eye contact that the patient makes with you; the depressed patient may be reluctant to look you in the eye. Also note the patient's general behaviour: is the person restless, does he or she appear anxious, are his or her movements retarded?

Speech

You may have noticed abnormalities during the interview: it is important to note them as they are indicators of psychological and neurological functioning. Note both the quantity and quality of the patient's speech. The patient who is depressed may speak in a slow, flat tone; the excitable, manic patient may have a rapid, pressurised way of speaking.

Mood

During the interview, you will have gathered information about mood or affect from the patient's behaviour and manner of expression. Does the patient seem depressed, anxious, agitated, manic or withdrawn? To explore this further, you can ask general questions, such as:

"I'm wondering if you still enjoy life as much as you used to?"

"How have you reacted to the problems you've had?"

"Perhaps you can tell me if you've felt a bit down (stressed, anxious, excited) recently."

Thought content

This refers to the patient's main concern, e.g. whether the patient has delusions or ideas about suicide. An appropriate first question would be: 'Could you tell me what's on your mind at present?' If the patient is obviously emotionally distressed, you should sensitively question about suicidal intent:

"You seem to have been having a lot of problems. I wonder if you sometimes think that life is not worth living?"

Cognitive function

This refers to the patient's orientation and general mental functioning. The preceding part of the interview will provide valuable clues as to whether the patient is oriented. If there is some doubt, an appropriate question would be: 'I'd like to ask you some questions about your thinking and memory. Could you tell me today's date and where you are now?' Tests of cognitive function include short-term memory tests, e.g. 'I'm going to tell you the names of three objects and I want you to remember them. The objects are fish, stars, house'. You can then ask the patient to recall the objects later in the interview. Another formal test is to ask the patient to subtract 7 from 100 continuously. By carrying out one such simple assessment of the patient's mental status, you will have a good idea of whether you should proceed with a more detailed examination of the patient's mental state at some stage of the interview.

Past medical history

Information about the patient's previous illnesses is important for an understanding of the presenting illness and management. You should obtain information about the patient's:

- previous general health
- previous illnesses
- admissions to hospital
- operations
- accidents and injuries
- pregnancies.

Begin by explaining what you intend to do, and then go through the topics you need to cover:

DR ROSS: *You've told me a lot about the problems you've had with your bowels, and I've asked you a number of questions. Now I'd like to ask you about any illnesses you've had in the past. Could you tell me about these?*

MRS ALTON: *Let me think, I had my appendix out when I was 15 or 16 and I had a chest infection when I was on holiday in the USA 5 years ago. That's all.*

DR ROSS: *Have you had any other operations?*

MRS ALTON: *No, I haven't.*

DR ROSS: *And have you been in hospital at any other time?*

MRS ALTON: *Only when I had the two children – they're grown up now.*

DR ROSS: *And did you have any problems with your pregnancies?*

MRS ALTON: *No – never felt better!*

DR ROSS: *Could you tell me if you've had any accidents or injured yourself at any time?*

MRS ALTON: *Well, yes. I slipped on the ice and broke my leg about 10 years ago. Actually I was in hospital then for several weeks – I'd forgotten that.*

DR ROSS: *Did they operate?*

MRS ALTON: *Yes, they did because they said it was a nasty break.*

DR ROSS: *OK, so just to summarise what you've told me: you had your appendix out when you were young and, more recently, you broke your leg and had a chest infection, but recovered well on each occasion.*

There are a number of specific conditions that you may want to exclude from the patient's past medical history at this stage. These will depend on circumstances but may include tuberculosis, rheumatic fever and diabetes.

You will notice that Dr Ross uses mainly closed questions because he wants specific information. It may be necessary to keep the patient to the point in this part of the interview: you need the bare bones of the patient's past history, unless it is relevant to the presenting complaint. Note that Dr Ross summarises what Mrs Alton tells him.

Family history

This is important for two reasons. First, the patient may be suffering from a genetically determined disease. Second, the patient's concerns about the presenting problems may be related to the experience of other members of the family. For example, Mrs Alton may be worried about her bowel symptoms because her father died from cancer of the colon. This is an important piece of information, partly because it will help you to interpret how she presents her symptoms and also because she has an increased risk of developing cancer of the colon, which is, at least in part, genetically determined.

When taking a family history ask about all first-degree relatives (parents, siblings, children), if they are living, and if not, the cause of death:

DR ROSS: *I'm sorry to hear that your father died of cancer. How old was he when he died?*
MRS ALTON: *He was 56, I think.*
DR ROSS: *And your mother?*
MRS ALTON: *Oh, she's well, apart from a bit of arthritis – she's 80.*

Taking a family history must be done sensitively. Patients will realise the importance of it if you explain the possible significance of the information. Towards the end, ask if there is a family history of specific diseases, e.g. heart disease, high blood pressure, diabetes. You may wish to draw a medical family tree (Fig. 3.5).

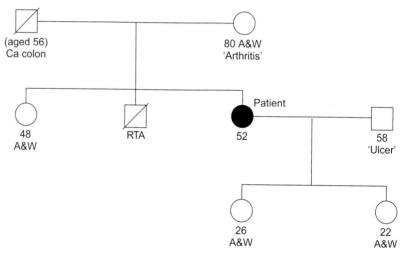

Fig. 3.5 Family tree of Mrs Alton. Ca, cancer; RTA, road traffic accident; A&W, alive and well.

Social history

In this part of the interview you should aim to build up a picture of the patient as a person outside the hospital or consulting room:

● How does the patient spend an average day?
● What is the structure of the patient's family and how do the members relate to each other?
● What is the patient's lifestyle?
● Does the patient have any worries about finance, accommodation, etc.?

This information will help you not only to interpret the way in which patients present their problems, but also to discuss the management of their problems. The social history can be conveniently divided into the patient profile, lifestyle (particularly risk factors) and sources of both stress and support.

Patient profile

This includes information about family life, other close relationships, work and daily activities. Suitable opening questions would be:

"Could you tell me something about yourself as a person? Perhaps you could start with your family and other people you are close to."

"Could you tell me what you do in an average day?"

You could conclude the personal profile by asking another open question: 'Is there anything else you think I should know about you and your family that would help me to understand you better?'

Occupational history

An occupational history is important because it may be of aetiological significance (e.g. hand dermatitis in people using strong detergents, back pain in nurses), or it may influence the ability to return to work (e.g. a nurse with back pain may be unable to return to her job in a geriatric ward). The essential features of an occupational history are:

● current job (what it involves, possible health hazards, how long in job, work-related stress)
● all previous jobs (details, and time in jobs).

Lifestyle

The patient's smoking and drinking habits are particularly important because they are risk factors for a number of diseases. You should aim to gather the following information:

Smoking history

Do you smoke? What do you smoke? How much do you smoke? How long have you smoked like this? If the patient is a non-smoker, ask if the patient smoked in the past and if so, for how long?

Drinking history

You may feel diffident about asking for details of alcohol consumption, but it is rare for a patient to resist if questioned appropriately. If the patient drinks, ask what and how much during an average week:

DR BUCK: *I'd like to ask you now about your drinking habits. Can you tell me if you drink alcohol?*
MR DAWES: *Yes, but not much. I suppose you'd call it social drinking.*
DR BUCK: *Could you tell me what you drink?*
MR DAWES: *Mostly beer: I go down to the pub most nights to have a few pints with my mates.*

DR BUCK: *A few pints? It would help me if you could go over the past week and give me an idea of how much you drank each evening.*

MR DAWES: *Well, let me see – I went down to the pub perhaps four times last week and drank about three pints each evening.*

DR BUCK: *Thank you, that's very helpful.*

You should record alcohol consumption in number of units per week. One unit is equivalent to the 8 grams of alcohol that is found in half a pint of beer, a small glass of wine (125 ml) or one pub measure of spirits. So Mr Dawes drank 24 units in the week before he saw Dr Buck.

Drug history
Include all current drugs prescribed by a doctor, all drugs that the patient has bought over the counter and recreational drugs if used.

Sources of stress

Health can be severely affected by stress related to work, personal relationships, finances and accommodation, so it is important to find out about these. Appropriate questions would be:

"Could you tell me if you feel particularly stressed?"

"What sort of things cause you stress?"

It is also important to find out about the sources of support that the patient may have: 'Perhaps you could tell me who you can turn to for support?'

By now you will be approaching the end of the interview and should be familiar with the patient's story and ready to write up your notes. As discussed in Chapter 2, the way in which you finish the interview is important. Remember the key features of closing an interview: summarise what you have been told; ask if the patient has any corrections, or additional information; and thank the patient for talking to you.

Writing up the patient's notes

Patients are likely to have told you their story in a way that does not fit neatly into the history-taking sequence. Writing up the notes enables you to organise the information. The notes should be written clearly and concisely under the same headings used for taking the patient's history (Table 3.1). Finish by summarising the most important points, listing the possible diagnoses and suggesting a management plan. When your notes are not going to be included in the patient's records, you should avoid including details that would allow someone else to identify the person, just in case your notes are lost. The easiest way of doing this is to use the patient's initials rather than full name.

The writing and keeping of notes are discussed in more detail in Chapter 12.

Can patients have access to their notes?

The answer is generally 'yes'. Under the Data Protection Act of 1998,[2] which came into force in March 2000, patients have the right of access to the information that a hospital or general practice holds about them. This applies to all paper and electronically held records. In exceptional circumstances access may be denied, for example when it is considered that a patient may be harmed by seeing his or her notes. It follows that you should never write anything that you would not wish the patient to see. It is now becoming common practice to send patients copies of the letters written about them and evidence shows that the majority would welcome this. This is discussed further in Chapter 12.

Modifying the history-taking sequence

It is important to learn and practise the history-taking sequence. By taking a history in a structured way you are less likely to miss important information. However, you will need to modify what you do in some situations. For example, it would be inappropriate to spend time taking a full medical history in casualty from a patient who has sustained a compound fracture of his leg in a road-traffic accident, or from a patient admitted with acute chest pain.

When you work in outpatient clinics and general practice you will notice that the doctor rarely takes a complete history when interviewing a patient. This reflects the way in which the doctor approaches the task of making a diagnosis and deciding on management. Gathering all possible information from a patient (history, physical examination and investigations), and only then working out the diagnosis, is not the most efficient way to make clinical decisions.

How then do doctors decide what is wrong with patients and how to manage them? Studies have shown that, early in an interview, doctors think of possible diagnoses (or hypotheses), based on clinical knowledge and experience. They then seek information from the patient that will either support or make unlikely each possible diagnosis. This process of clinical decision-making (called the hypothetico-deductive method) develops with experience. You will find yourself beginning to postulate diagnoses whilst taking a history and these will influence the way in which you ask further questions. But remember, you must establish a firm clinical base for yourself by learning to take a systematic history.

The medical interview and the Cambridge–Calgary guides

In this chapter we have covered the fundamentals of the medical interview and in the next chapter we shall discuss how to give information. In Chapter 2 we outlined the basic skills of good communication; the

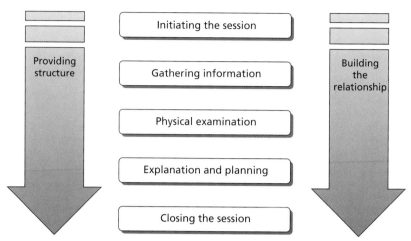

Fig. 3.6 Cambridge–Calgary guide basic framework. © Kurtz S, Silverman J, Draper J (eds) 2005 Teaching and learning communication skills in medicine. Radcliffe Publishing, Oxford. Reproduced with the permission of the copyright holder.

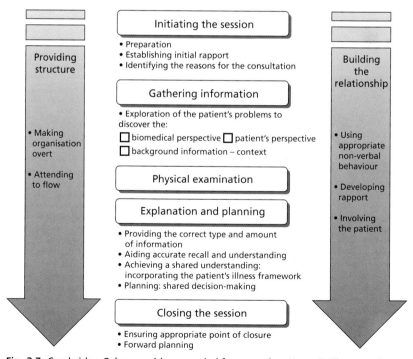

Fig. 3.7 Cambridge-Calgary guide expanded framework. © Kurtz S, Silverman J, Draper J (eds) 2005 Teaching and learning communication skills in medicine. Radcliffe Publishing, Oxford. Reproduced with the permission of the copyright holder.

way in which we use these skills is the *process* component of the interview. The information gathered as the medical history and given to the patient during the explanation phase is the *content* component of the interview. The integration of these two components is often difficult and confusing, particularly for students at the beginning of their training. In an attempt to facilitate their integration, Jonathan Silverman and his colleagues designed the Cambridge–Calgary guides[3] which are now widely used in both teaching and research. The basic framework, which includes the physical examination, is shown in Figure 3.6 and the more detailed framework in Figure 3.7. You will notice that the headings in the horizontal bars are parts of the interview to be dealt with in sequence and those in the vertical bars are the aspects of the interview which you need to attend to throughout the interview.

Some practical hints for taking a history

- Take every opportunity you are given to interview patients. You will only develop the skills through repeated practice. Books like this one will be helpful, but they are no substitute for patients.
- Be prepared to spend time with patients – this is necessary in order to learn how to take an accurate, systematic history. You will speed up as you become more experienced.
- You are more likely to obtain a good history if you use the skills outlined in Chapter 2:
  - Establish rapport.
  - Listen actively.
  - Ask mainly open questions.
  - Pick up and respond to verbal and non-verbal cues.
  - Facilitate or help if the patient gets stuck.
  - Summarise and check for accuracy.
- Make an aide-mémoire of the history-taking sequence.
- Most people need to take notes as they are interviewing. You may decide to make rough notes and to write them up later. Remember to explain why you are taking notes and check if it is acceptable. Always maintain intermittent eye contact, and don't give the impression that your notes are more important than what the patient is saying.

Presenting a patient at a ward round

Presenting a patient at a case conference or ward round is an integral part of traditional medical education. At first, all students are likely to find this a daunting experience that may provoke anxiety. However, even if practice does not ensure perfection, it should increase your confidence and competence (Table 3.2).

Table 3.2 Guidelines for presenting a patient on a ward round

Preparation
- Obtain as much information as possible from your patient, i.e. the history, the findings on physical examination and results of investigations
- Identify the most important features you wish to emphasise
- Think about possible questions you might be asked
- Read up in a textbook about the patient's condition
- Summarise details using headings and write them down (aide-mémoire)

Presentation
- Relax
- Speak clearly and fluently
- Be concise
- Be accurate
- If you are asked questions and know the answer, express it confidently; if you are unsure or do not know, it is probably best to say so
- Be sensitive to the needs of the patient if he or she is present

Follow up
- If possible, go back to see your patient after the round to discuss any concerns he or she may have arising from what he or she heard
- Reflect on your presentation. What did you do well? What could you have improved? Ask for feedback from your peers

---

Let us look at the purposes of presenting patients at ward rounds or conferences:

- On ward rounds particularly, the consultant and other medical and nursing staff can learn about the patient's history and the findings of the physical examination and investigation. As a student, you are likely to have had the time to get to know your patient well, to have obtained a history and to have carried out a physical examination.
- The presentation of a patient will stimulate discussion on diagnosis and management.
- It is an important learning opportunity for students. Presenting information to others is a crucial skill to be acquired in training and something you will have to do throughout your professional life.

Common concerns about interviewing patients

The patient refuses to see me

This rarely happens. Most patients are happy to see students and often benefit from the time and support you may be able to give them. Sometimes, however, a patient may have told his or her story to several students and does not want to do it again. Don't take refusal to see you as a personal affront.

I forget what question to ask next

Remember that interviewing a patient involves more than asking questions. It is natural to feel anxious when there are gaps in the conversation, but silences are important. If you lose the thread of the interview, you might carry on by summarising what the patient has told you so far.

The patient asks me a question about his or her condition

As a general rule, you should not answer questions that patients may ask you about their condition but suggest that they ask their doctor. Clearly, you will have to use your own judgement. If the patient asks you a simple factual question and you are confident of the answer, you might reply, but never be afraid to say, 'I don't know, but I'll ask Dr Peters to discuss this with you', or, 'I don't know. I'll go and look it up'.

The patient tells me something in confidence

Confidentiality of information is an essential part of the patient–doctor relationship and has been enshrined in professional codes of practice since Hippocrates. Patients may feel that it is easier to talk to you as a student, particularly as you may be able to spend more time with them than the rest of the staff. Occasionally, a patient may give you information that he or she asks you to keep confidential. This puts you in a difficult position, particularly if the information is pertinent to the patient's management. Some general guidelines are:

● Only in very exceptional circumstances should a doctor break a patient's confidence when the patient has not given consent for information to be divulged.
● As a student never promise a patient confidentiality.
● Explore why the patient feels he or she can't discuss it with a member of the medical team. This may help the patient to realise he or she should tell the doctor if it is relevant to the condition and treatment.
● If in doubt, discuss your predicament with a senior member of staff, without divulging the information given you.

The patient starts crying or becomes emotional

It is natural to feel anxious and embarrassed when a patient breaks down in tears. Try to control your anxiety (it may be communicated to the patient), avoid rushing in with questions and give the patient an opportunity to express emotion. You can help the patient to do this through empathy, perhaps by touching the patient's hand, or using reflective comments:

"I understand that this must be very upsetting for you."

"I can understand why you are so upset."

"Perhaps you would like to tell me more about how you feel."

Key points

■ It is important to obtain a complete and accurate history: for the majority of patients, a diagnosis can be made on the history alone.
■ Develop and practise a systematic approach to taking a history:
 – introduction and explanation of task
 – personal details
 – presenting problem(s)
 – history of presenting problem(s)
 – review of body systems
 – past medical history
 – family history
 – social history
 – summarise and conclude interview.
■ Good communication skills are essential. Use open questions, listen carefully, and pick up and respond to verbal and non-verbal cues.

FURTHER READING

Bradley G W 1993 Disease, diagnosis and decisions. John Wiley, Chichester

Noble LM 2007 Written communication. In: Ayers S, Baum A, McManus C et al (eds) Psychology, health and medicine. Cambridge University Press, Cambridge

Silverman J, Kurtz S, Draper J 2005 Skills for communicating with patients, 2nd edn. Radcliffe Medical Publishing, Oxford

REFERENCES

1. Hampton JR, Harrison MJG, Mitchell JRA et al 1975 Relative contribution of history-taking, physical examination, and laboratory investigation to diagnosis and management of medical outpatients. British Medical Journal 2: 486–489

2. Data Protection Act 1998 Available online at: www.legislation.hmso.gov.uk

3. Kurtz S, Silverman J, Draper J 2005 Teaching and learning communication skills in medicine, 2nd edn. Radcliffe Medical Publishing, Oxford

4

Giving information

In the last chapter we concentrated on how to gather information from a patient. This, together with the information obtained from the physical examination and investigations, will enable a diagnosis to be made for most patients, and a management plan to be devised for all patients. At some point, perhaps in the same interview or perhaps in a subsequent one, there will be a need to explain and discuss what has been found and what investigations and treatment are planned. It is important to remember that most treatments involve the cooperation of the patient – providing, of course, the patient is capable of cooperation. The way in which information is given has been shown in a number of studies to have a major effect on several aspects of patient care, including:

- Patients' level of anxiety and stress: this has been shown to decrease if patients are given adequate information prior to investigations and surgical procedures.
- The outcome of these procedures: there is some evidence to suggest that patients who are given a full explanation of the operation they are about to undergo spend less time in hospital and require fewer pain-relieving drugs than patients who have not been fully informed.
- Satisfaction with care: patients who are given a full explanation of their problem and its management in a way which they understand are more likely to be satisfied with their care. This is desirable in itself, but there is also evidence that a satisfied patient is more likely to comply with advice than someone who is dissatisfied.
- Compliance with treatment: patients are more likely to comply with their treatment if they are satisfied with their consultation and if they understand why they have to undergo the treatment.

Unfortunately, doctors are not very good at giving information to patients. Failure to give information or adequate explanation is the most common cause of dissatisfaction amongst patients. Here are some quotes from patients included in a report on communication between hospitals and patients:[1]

"You have to fight to be told what's wrong"
(patient who had had a stroke).

"Why is it that no one wants to discuss it? It wouldn't hurt to know the side-effects of drugs"
(patient with rheumatoid arthritis).

"I didn't even know if it was malignant...perhaps they leave it to your imagination"
(woman with breast cancer).

STOP AND THINK   *Think of the possible reasons why these patients did not get the information they wanted.*

There is evidence from a number of studies that the way in which doctors give information to patients is inadequate.[2] First, patients often do not remember the information they are given. In one study in an outpatient clinic, it was found that patients had forgotten 40% of the information within 2 hours of seeing the doctor. This rose to 54% when patients were asked to recall the information 1–4 weeks after the consultation. Second, patients often do not follow the advice given. Several studies have found that 30–50% of patients do not take their drugs as prescribed.

An article in the *British Medical Journal* entitled 'Most young doctors are bad at giving information' described a study of doctors who had received training in interviewing skills when they were students.[3] Whilst their ability to gather information from the patient remained high, their ability to give information had not, and the majority were thought to have performed inadequately. What are the possible explanations for these findings? The explanations concern the processes involved in exchanging information.

The person giving the information

To give information effectively, you must:

- understand the information and be able to convey it accurately
- use ideas and language that the listener can understand
- be prepared to respond to the recipient's questions and emotional reaction.

The person receiving the information

- The recipient should be able to listen to and concentrate on what is said. We are less likely to listen and remember if we are tired or anxious, or have symptoms such as pain or nausea.
- Patients will remember the information more easily if they are able to link it to their existing knowledge, if it has been reinforced during the interview and if they are asked to review what has been said.

Clearly, there are skills involved in giving information that doctors may not be aware of. First, there is more to it than simply telling patients what is wrong and what they should do. Second, it is often wrongly assumed that patients are not capable of understanding explanations of their medical problems because of lack of knowledge. Third, it is often assumed that patients are made more anxious if the details of their problem and its management are explained to them. There is no evidence that this is so. Lack of information and uncertainty about their diagnosis and treatment are more likely to increase anxiety. There is considerable evidence now that most patients want to know what is wrong with them, even if the news is not good. Giving patients this information has a positive effect on them – providing, of course, it is given in a manner sensitive to their needs.

How to give information

So what are the skills involved in giving information to patients? First of all, think about the aims you wish to achieve:

- To help the patient understand what is happening
- To reduce the patient's anxiety and uncertainty as far as possible
- To gain the patient's cooperation in the management of the problem.

To achieve these aims, you must first find out what the patient understands about the problem and how the patient thinks he or she might be helped. Then, you need to tailor the information you give accordingly.

Guidelines for giving information to a patient (Table 4.1)

Table 4.1 Giving information to a patient

1. Describe what information you plan to give
2. Summarise your understanding of the patient's problems
3. Find out the patient's understanding of the condition
4. Outline the structure of the rest of the interview
5. Use appropriate language
6. If relevant, use drawings to supplement the information
7. Give the most important piece of information first
8. Explore the patient's views on the information given
9. Negotiate management
10. Check the patient's understanding of what has been said

1. Describe what information you plan to give

Clarify in your own mind the information you plan to give. This will probably fall into the following categories:

- results of the physical examination
- results of tests
- diagnosis (or provisional diagnosis)

- cause of the problems
- necessary further investigations
- treatment planned
- prognosis
- advice about lifestyle.

2. Summarise your understanding of the patient's problems

Begin the interview by summarising the patient's problems (the information gathered to date):

> DR SMITH: *You've told me about the pain in your stomach and the heartburn you've been having after meals and at night. You also mentioned that you've had an ulcer in the past. Is that right?*
>
> MR BARNES: *Yes – they found I had an ulcer when I was serving in the army – about 10 years ago.*

3. Find out the patient's understanding of the condition

Assess the patient's understanding of the condition:

> DR SMITH: *Could you tell me what you think is causing your symptoms?*
> *or*
>
> DR SMITH: *Most people have some ideas or worries about what is causing the problem. Do you have any ideas?*
>
> MR BARNES: *Well, I think my ulcer's come back because of my new job – driving a lorry up to Scotland and back. I'm a bit worried because my friend got peritonitis from a burst ulcer.*

4. Outline the structure of the rest of the interview

Outline how you plan to structure the rest of the interview. You may plan to discuss the diagnosis, treatment and future investigations. It has been shown that structuring the interview and explaining what you plan to discuss improves the patient's recall of the information given:

> DR SMITH: *Fine, I understand. Now I'm going to discuss several things with you: first, what I think is wrong with you; second, what further investigations you need; and lastly, the treatment I'm going to give you.*

5. Use appropriate language

Describe and explain each part of the information. In doing this, it is important to:

- give the most important information first
- use short words and short sentences
- avoid medical jargon
- be specific – vague information only increases anxiety.

It is all too easy to use words and medical phrases familiar to you but which the patient will not understand. When you use them, ask if the patient understands.

DR SMITH: *Well, your barium meal did not show an ulcer. But it did show that you have something we call a hiatus hernia. Do you know what that is?*

MR BARNES: *I think my grandmother had one, but I haven't much of a clue, really.*

6. If relevant, use drawings to supplement the information

In the above case, Dr Smith could explain a hiatus hernia to Mr Barnes much more easily using drawings than using words.

7. Give the most important piece of information first

This is particularly necessary when giving advice:

DR SMITH: *Now, I'm going to explain how we can try to get rid of your symptoms. I think it would help if you were able to lose a bit of weight. You will be less likely to get the pain if you can eat smaller meals regularly. For example, instead of one large meal at night, I suggest you eat a good breakfast (such as cereal or toast), perhaps a light lunch, such as sandwiches, and then have your evening meal, which should be smaller than usual. I suggest that you sleep on three pillows because then the acid in your stomach is less likely to come up into your gullet than when you lie flat. Lastly, I'm going to give you some tablets that will stop your stomach producing acid; you should take one each morning.*

8. Explore the patient's views on the information given

Encourage the patient to ask questions:

DR SMITH: *Perhaps you could tell me what you feel about that.*

MR BARNES: *Well, I'm really surprised that I haven't got an ulcer because my pain felt just the same as last time. But yes, I understand what a hiatus hernia is now that you've drawn one. I'm worried that it might be difficult for me to eat the meals you suggest because I'm on the road most of the day, and I'm not sure if I want to take those tablets.*

9. Negotiate management

Negotiate management with the patient. If appropriate, help the patient to decide between treatment options:

DR SMITH: *Yes, I understand you might have some problems with the diet I'm suggesting, especially as roadside cafés usually sell lots of greasy food. However, perhaps you could keep to the*

> *fish and chicken and avoid the chips and fried eggs. You say you're not keen on taking tablets – why not?*
>
> MR BARNES: *A friend of mine had them and then he got worse, and 6 weeks later they found he had stomach cancer.*
>
> DR SMITH: *I see. So are you worried about having cancer?*
>
> MR BARNES: *I was, a bit. I suppose if my X-ray only showed a hernia, I must be clear. Are there other tests you can do to be absolutely sure?*
>
> DR SMITH: *Yes, there are, but I don't think it's necessary to do them at present. We'll want to see how you get on over the next few weeks with a change of diet. What about the tablets I've suggested? I don't think it's possible that they caused your friend's cancer.*
>
> MR BARNES: *I think I'd rather try changing my diet first of all and taking the white medicine you prescribed for me last time.*
>
> DR SMITH: *Let's try that for the next 4 weeks, then I'll see you again.*

Note that Dr Smith does not elicit Mr Barnes's fear of cancer until this stage of the interview. Once out in the open, Dr Smith acknowledges Mr Barnes's concerns and takes them into account during the rest of the interview. He also gives Mr Barnes the opportunity to express his treatment preference. Eventually, they decide on a treatment plan that is acceptable to both, and one that Mr Barnes is likely to follow because he was involved in making the decision.

10. Check the patient's understanding of what has been said

Check understanding:

> DR SMITH: *Well, Mr Barnes, I seem to have given you lots of information. Would you like to go over what we have said?*

Giving lifestyle advice

Doctors are increasingly being asked to help patients modify aspects of their lifestyle that may be hazardous to their health. Smoking, excessive drinking, lack of exercise, a high-fat diet and unsafe sex are all examples of behaviours that carry a health risk. In the general practice setting, the emphasis is on helping patients to reduce their risks of developing disease, e.g. by stopping smoking. In the hospital setting, the emphasis may be more on helping patients with established disease to adopt behaviours that reduce disability or the chance of a recurrence.

As a medical student, you may be asked by patients, 'How can I give up smoking?' In the past, it was thought that if patients were given information, e.g. about the hazards of smoking and how to stop, then their knowledge about smoking would increase and this would lead to a change in their attitudes and behaviour. We now realise that helping patients to change involves more than just providing them with information.

Case example 4.1

A habitual smoker with asthma

Mr O'Shea, aged 52, is an unemployed man admitted with an acute asthmatic attack.

DR SINGH: *Well, Mr O'Shea, you're much better now and it's time to go home. I've seen you a few times in the day room smoking – you shouldn't be doing that with a chest like yours. I think I've told you that before. Make sure you've stopped by the time I see you next in the outpatient clinic. Smoking does terrible things to your chest, you know.*

MR O'SHEA: *OK, doctor, I'll try.*

Four weeks later in the outpatient clinic:

DR SINGH: *Hello, Mr O'Shea. So how is your asthma? I hope you've given up smoking!*

MR O'SHEA: *My asthma's not too bad – except some mornings when my chest feels really tight and I'm up all night coughing sometimes. I sort of tried to give up smoking but didn't manage it.*

DR SINGH: *So how many are you smoking?*

MR O'SHEA: *Still 20 a day – sometimes a bit less.*

STOP AND THINK 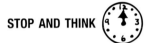 *Mr O'Shea did not heed Dr Singh's advice to stop smoking. Are you surprised? Think about other approaches that Dr Singh could have adopted within the interview that might have been more successful.*

How to give lifestyle advice

This process can be divided into four stages. We will use the example of advising a patient to give up smoking.

Stage 1: enquire about the patient's attitudes to health

This will help you to understand why the patient smokes and to tailor your advice accordingly. An American social psychologist has proposed a health belief model that can be summarised as the three Ss:

- *Susceptibility*: how does the person perceive his or her vulnerability to a particular disease? A person who has a strong family history of smoking and early deaths from cardiovascular disease is likely to view his or her susceptibility differently, and may be more motivated to give up, compared to someone whose grandparents and parents smoked heavily and lived to a ripe old age.
- *Seriousness*: how does the individual perceive the seriousness of the consequences of developing or exacerbating a particular disease? In the case example, to what extent does Mr O'Shea believe that his asthma is made worse by smoking?

- *Solutions*: how does the person weigh the costs and benefits of a particular course of action, such as giving up smoking? Smokers may want to accept the financial and potential health costs of smoking because they enjoy it and feel that it relieves their stress.

Stage 2: giving information

Having obtained an understanding of the patient's attitudes to the problem, you are in a better position to provide information about smoking and how to stop.

Remember some basic rules about giving information:

- Organise the information into categories and explain what they are.
- Give instruction and advice early in the interview.
- Make the advice specific.
- Use short words and short sentences.
- Avoid medical jargon.
- Repeat the advice during the course of the interview.

Stage 3: negotiating

It is important to negotiate a plan of action with the patient. Find out if the patient is still firmly committed to stopping smoking; if so, what does the individual feel is an achievable, realistic target? This should be discussed and a plan of action agreed. Remember to ask the patient to summarise what has been agreed so that you can check the patient's understanding of the plan.

Stage 4: supporting the patient

Changing one's lifestyle – such as giving up a lifelong habit of smoking or drinking – is not easy, and continued support should be given. The plan of action that has been negotiated should be reviewed and may need to be renegotiated at intervals.

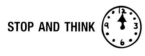

STOP AND THINK

Re-read the case example of Mr O'Shea and Dr Singh. How might Dr Singh have conducted the interview more effectively, bearing in mind the guidelines you have just read? You might want to create a role-play of Mr O'Shea and Dr Singh.

The use of written information

A number of studies have shown that patients want information in the form of pamphlets or booklets, and that they benefit from written information.[4] Such material can supplement verbal explanation and advice, provide a permanent record and cover all the important points to be conveyed to the patient. Evidence shows that written information, presented in an appropriate form, enhances patients' understanding and memory. Written information should be:

- easy to read – use short words and sentences
- expressed in the active rather that the passive voice, i.e. 'we think' instead of 'it is thought'
- expressed in positive rather than negative sentences
- attractively presented.

It seems likely that, in the next decade, electronic means of conveying information will overtake the printed word. Some general practitioners are now using videos in their waiting rooms to provide patients with information. Interactive videos are being used, not only to provide information, but also to involve patients in decision-making. For example, male patients with benign prostatic hypertrophy are being helped to decide whether or not to have an operation by means of a video that they can interact with.

Obtaining informed consent

All patients who are assessed as being competent must give their consent before any procedure is carried out on them. This includes physical examination. Without it, a doctor can be legally charged with assault. Recently, the need to gain consent from patients when they are involved in teaching has been highlighted.[5] In particular, all patients must give their written consent to rectal and vaginal examinations by students when they are sedated or anaesthetised.

One of a house surgeon's jobs is to obtain patients' informed consent in writing before they undergo any surgical procedure. In the UK the standard consent form includes the sentence: 'I confirm that I have explained to the patient the nature and purpose of this operation'. The doctor signs below, and the patient signs to confirm that: 'the nature and purpose of the operation have been explained to me by Dr . . .'.

Concern is often raised as to whether or not the patient's consent is truly 'informed'. The issues that need to be addressed are the nature of the information given to the patient, the manner in which it is given and the way in which consent is obtained. Here are some guidelines for obtaining informed consent from a patient:[6]

1. The patient should be given information about the procedure, its benefits and risks. The nature of the operation should be clearly explained, perhaps with the aid of a drawing, if appropriate. Then the benefits and possible risks should be discussed.[7] One of the dilemmas is how much information should be given about the risks. On the one hand, we do not want to alarm the patient by itemising all the possible risks (some of which may be very remote), but on the other hand, the patient needs to be fully informed. It is difficult to give hard and fast rules. It is clearly important to encourage the patient to ask questions and to give clear, truthful answers.
2. It is essential that the patient understands the information. This means following the rules of information-giving:

    a. Explain how you are going to structure the information: 'First of all, I'm going to explain what the surgeon will do. Then we will discuss how we think it will help you. Lastly, I will talk about the problems which could arise.'

    b. Use short words and short sentences.

    c. Avoid medical jargon.

    d. Check the patient's understanding of what you have said.

    e. Does the patient have any questions?

    f. Does the patient give consent for the procedure?

    Adequate time must be allowed for this process. It might be tempting to think of it as a quick formality at the end of clerking of the patient. Quite apart from the legal aspects, it has been shown that patients who are fully informed are more satisfied and may make a better postoperative recovery.

3. The patient's consent must be given voluntarily and no coercion must be used. Remember that there are subtle ways of putting pressure on someone who has to make a decision, and these must be avoided.

4. The patient must be considered competent to sign the form. This means that you have judged the patient capable of understanding the information given, and that the patient is able to make a choice and able to communicate it to you. If you are not sure that the patient is able to satisfy these criteria, the patient's capacity to give consent should be formally assessed.[8] Further guidance on how this should be done is set out in the Mental Capacity Act 2005.[9]

We have discussed informed consent in the context of a patient about to undergo surgery. There are, of course, other circumstances in which it will be necessary to obtain consent (taking part in a research project, for example), but the same procedure should be followed.

    Obtaining informed consent is important for the patient and the doctor. It is not a task to be taken lightly, and it is a good test of your ability to convey information effectively and sensitively.

Key points

- The way in which information is given influences patients' satisfaction and compliance with treatment.
- Before giving information, find out what the patient knows about the problem and its possible treatment and take this into account when giving information.
- Outline the stages of giving the information (diagnosis, treatment, etc.).
- When giving information:
  - give the most important information first
  - use short words and short sentences
  - avoid medical jargon
  - avoid vagueness – give specific information.

- When deciding on a treatment plan with a patient:
  - identify and acknowledge the patient's beliefs and worries about the problem and its management
  - find out the patient's treatment preference
  - negotiate a treatment plan.
- At the end of the interview, ask the patient to summarise what has been agreed.

FURTHER READING

Ley P 1988 Communicating with patients: improving communication, satisfaction and compliance. Chapman & Hall, London

REFERENCES

1. Audit Commission 1993 'What seems to be the matter?': communication between hospitals and patients. HMSO, London
2. Silverman J, Kurtz SM, Draper J 2005 Skills for communicating with patients, 2nd edn. Radcliffe Publishing, Oxford
3. Maguire P, Fairbairn S, Fletcher C 1986 Consultation skills of young doctors: most young doctors are bad at giving information. British Medical Journal 292: 1576–1578
4. Noble LM 2007 Written communication. In: Ayers S, Baum A, McManus C et al (eds) Psychology, health and medicine. Cambridge University Press, Cambridge
5. Singer PA 2003 Intimate examinations and other ethical challenges in medical education. British Medical Journal 326: 62–63
6. Department of Health 2001 Good practice in consent implementation guide: consent to examination or treatment. Available online at: www.dh.gov.uk/consent
7. French DP, Marteau TM 2007 Communicating risk. In: Ayers S, Baum A, McManus C et al (eds) Psychology, health and medicine. Cambridge University Press, Cambridge
8. Nicholson TRJ, Cutter W, Hotopf M 2008 Assessing mental capacity: the Mental Capacity Act. British Medical Journal 336: 322–325
9. Mental Capacity Act 2005. Available online at: www.dca.gov.uk/legal-policy/mental-capacity/mca-cp.pdf

5

Breaking bad news

Breaking bad news is an inevitable part of medical practice. Most of us worry about our ability to communicate sensitive and sometimes distressing news to patients and their relatives. This is not altogether surprising, as the subject of breaking bad news is still not widely taught in medical schools, and only rarely is reference made to the topic in medical, surgical and psychiatric textbooks. Research has focused on how patients and their relatives cope with bad news, rather than on the process of breaking bad news. More is known about the psychological consequences of bad news than how best to deliver it. But we also know that what and how people are told affects their trust in their medical practitioner as well as how they cope and adjust in the future.

The trend towards increased openness in the relationship between doctors and their patients makes it important to focus attention in communications skills training on those procedures and hints that help us to deliver bad news. Most patients nowadays are not satisfied with patronising euphemisms and evasion. On the other hand, breaking bad news in a direct and abrupt manner, without taking into account the patient's need for information, can be damaging. There is an increasing recognition that bad news can be given tactfully and that the process can begin to prepare patients and relatives for what may be ahead. This chapter considers what bad news consists of, addresses why it is often difficult to break bad news and describes an approach to giving bad news that can be adapted for different settings, with different patients and in relation to a range of issues.

What is bad news?

  What would you consider bad news in your life? Finding out that you had failed an exam? Not getting the job you wanted? Hearing that a relative or someone close to you was ill or had died? Being refused a bank loan? How was the bad news given to you? Directly, in a roundabout way, in a letter or over the phone? What was your first reaction? How did you cope? Did you feel differently about the news 3 hours later? The next day? Could the news have been given to you differently, or in a way that softened the blow?

The death of a patient or the diagnosis of serious illness, progressive disease or handicap is usually considered bad news. Some doctors would add having to tell a patient that there is no bed available in the hospital, that the patient's medical notes have been misplaced or that an operation has had to be cancelled. Conventionally, the concept pertains to situations where there is a feeling of no hope, a threat to an individual's mental and physical well-being, a risk of upsetting an established lifestyle, or where a message is given which implies the person has fewer choices in life. It may be tempting to consider whether news is good or bad for an individual. Some people, when diagnosed with a terminal illness, cope with the news, yet for others, minor ailments that are treatable can be distressing and are interpreted as signs of bad news. News, of whatever kind, is information, whereas the idea that it is either good or bad is a belief, value judgement or affective response from either the provider or the receiver of the information.

There are many situations in which doctors might preface giving news with 'I am sorry to tell you that ...', or 'I am pleased to tell you ...', illustrating how value and meaning are attached to information from the outset. Such preconceptions about what is good and bad news are based on personal and professional experience. However, in some cases, these preconceptions may directly influence a patient's emotional responses to this information. A patient who is given so-called good news in the form of a negative HIV antibody test result may feel ashamed to cry or discuss new problems. For that patient, for example, there may be an element of bad news, as he or she then feels that there are no excuses for failing in a sexual relationship, whereas previously the fear of HIV had been a protection from meeting new partners. Similarly, a patient who feels some relief about an AIDS diagnosis may be concerned that the doctor may misconstrue this as denial, emotional blunting or suggestive of psychiatric disorder.

Bad news is, therefore, a relative concept and should depend on the patient's interpretation of information and reaction to it. Where patients feel the news will adversely affect their future, then it can be considered bad news. Usually, we can predict what will be viewed as bad news, but not with complete certainty. Clinical experience highlights the value of sometimes waiting until the patient attaches new meaning to the information before defining it as good or bad news. This does not mean that we are unaffected by patients' feelings and responses, but that we should try to avoid making assumptions as to what these may be, and not inhibit patients' reactions by our own.

What is difficult about giving bad news?

There are personal, professional and social reasons why giving bad news to patients may be difficult (Table 5.1). Training in medicine emphasises treatment, healing and the reduction of suffering. Serious illness, a deterioration in a patient's condition, handicap, disability or death

Table 5.1 Why is it difficult to give bad news?

- The 'messenger' may feel responsible and fears being blamed
- Not knowing how best to do it
- Possible inhibition because of personal experience of loss
- Reluctance to change the existing doctor–patient relationship
- Fear of upsetting the patient's existing family roles or structure
- Not knowing the patient, his or her resources and limitations
- Fear of the implications for the patient, e.g. disfigurement, pain, social and financial losses
- Fear of the patient's emotional reaction
- Uncertainty as to what may happen next and not having answers to some questions
- Lack of clarity about one's own role as a health care provider

all confront us with some of the limitations of modern medicine. In some situations, we may feel responsible for inflicting emotional pain or suffering on patients and their family. In the role of a messenger, we may fear being blamed, and experience personal failure. Bad news often implies the loss of well-being, youth, hope, health and relationships. We mark a transition in life for patients and their family that may be either premature or unwelcome, or both. The news ushers in new family roles: perhaps a partner becomes a carer or a widow, a generation may end in the family and all others may move up in the family structure. For the patient who is unwell, there is the sick role and the associated social stigma. Many people may fear disfigurement, physical pain, loneliness and infectiousness, as well as questions about emotional, social and financial well-being.

Doctors and other health care professionals themselves are not immune to the experience of personal loss. A recent experience of loss or illness in our own family may make it difficult for us to break bad news to our patients and to give them support. It may also be difficult to anticipate how a patient or relative might react, and this unpredictability may deter us from giving bad news. Some doctors worry that their own emotional reactions – such as wanting to cry – might make them appear unprofessional in the eyes of the patient.

Another reason for difficulty in giving bad news is a fear of extreme reactions, such as the threat of violence, emotional distress and suicidal thoughts. Other reasons for a reluctance to give bad news may be more subtle. Telling a patient he or she has a chronic condition, such as diabetes or haemophilia, means that person will have a lifelong relationship with the health care system. It may be difficult to countenance such a relationship with certain patients and, instead, we might delegate the task of giving the diagnosis to another doctor, such as a GP or hospital specialist. On the other hand, bad news may spell the end of a close professional relationship with a patient, and the personal loss may be difficult for us to face.

A fear of 'doing it wrong', or giving incorrect information, may also deter us. Lastly, the example of senior colleagues or one's own position as a professional in transition may make it difficult to know how to deal with a patient. A few consultants still hold the view that patients should not be told they are dying; this makes it difficult for a junior doctor to deal openly with the patient's expressed concerns and fears. Similarly, medical students sometimes report that patients ask them to confirm the diagnosis because the medical and nursing staff have not openly discussed it with them. Often this creates a dilemma for the student who may be privy to important information but not have the authority to talk about it openly with the patient.

Options for managing difficult situations

Before describing some guidelines for giving bad news, we need to consider what options may be available for managing difficult clinical situations. There are four main considerations, described below.

To whom should bad news be given?

Certain legal and ethical guidelines in clinical practice make it difficult for a doctor to choose to withhold important and personal information from the patient. It is almost impossible to justify doing so 'to protect the patient' or 'because it would hurt the patient to know'. Nonetheless, circumstances may arise where other specific factors may need to be taken into account before deciding to break bad news. It is good practice first to discuss these situations with a colleague or within a multidisciplinary health care team. There are some specific situations in which you may need to consider whether to give bad news. For example, if a patient is deemed to be psychotic, and presumably may not understand what has happened, there may be reason to withhold bad news. When treating a child, one usually confers with the parent or guardian before breaking bad news.

Who should give bad news?

For several reasons, it may be more appropriate for another doctor to break bad news. For example, a patient sent to a hospital for special tests may still expect his or her GP to reveal the results, rather than the hospital consultant. The GP usually has an established relationship with the patient and presumably could anticipate some of the problems that might arise. Giving bad news usually requires time, so it may be inappropriate for someone to do so at the end of a shift. It may be preferable to hand over the task to other colleagues, provided they are fully briefed and acquainted with the case. But it is poor practice to delegate the task to a colleague because you do not feel like confronting the patient yourself.

When should bad news be given?

Where patients are diagnosed as having a chronic or degenerative medical condition, or where an infant is born with a handicap that is not immediately apparent, there is usually the option of withholding the bad news until a later stage. One advantage is that you can try gradually to break the news; this in turn gives the patient and relatives time to adjust. On the other hand, withholding the news may deny them the opportunity to face up to it and begin to make the necessary adjustments in their personal lives.

In some situations, it can actually be hazardous to withhold bad news until a later stage. If the patient has an infectious disease or condition (e.g. hepatitis C or HIV infection), he or she can inadvertently infect someone else, or be denied the benefits of early medical information if not fully informed of this condition. A further disadvantage of withholding the news at an early stage is that when the patient becomes physically very unwell, he or she is less likely to have the emotional and practical resources to make the necessary adjustments (e.g. say goodbye to children, or settle financial matters). Of course, there are obviously some situations where there is no choice and bad news must be given immediately (e.g. informing relatives of a death).

Should you give hope and reassurance along with bad news?

You can reassure patients that their fears for the future are probably worse than the reality. This option may be difficult to resist because, by conveying hope, it can result in an immediate reduction of a patient's anxiety and distress. It is a form of emotional first aid that may be indicated where patients appear to be isolated and in extreme distress. However, reassurance is sometimes inappropriate and may serve to sweep fear under the carpet that will only resurface later on. Where doctors repeatedly reassure patients, they may take on some of their patients' anxiety and assume responsibility for some decisions that could otherwise be shared. This can lead to feelings of burnout and stress, and doctors also run the risk of colluding with patients' denial of the severity of problems, or potential problems, if false hope is offered.

How to give bad news

(p. 191) **Exercise 6** There are several practical and logical steps that can be followed when giving bad news (Table 5.2). Although these serve as guidelines, there are no firm rules for what is often one of the most challenging aspects of medical practice. It is always a matter of clinical judgement and professional experience as to how bad news should be broken, and each situation must be treated differently. There are five main considerations:

Table 5.2 The process of giving bad news

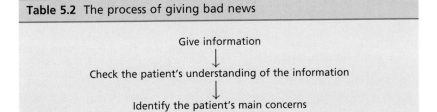

Give information

↓

Check the patient's understanding of the information

↓

Identify the patient's main concerns

↓

Elicit the patient's coping strategies and personal resources
and give realistic hope

1. personal preparation
2. the physical setting
3. talking to the patient and responding to concerns
4. arranging follow-up or referral
5. feedback and handover to colleagues.

Personal preparation

It takes time to give bad news properly and instil confidence and support by being available to answer questions. For this reason, it is not usually appropriate to break bad news in the middle of a busy clinic or during a ward round. Before seeing the patient, you should first take a few moments to consider what information is known and what needs to be addressed. The following points should be considered:

- Is the patient expecting bad news, or am I 'going in cold'?
- Should anyone else be present (such as a nurse or relative)?
- What does the patient already know about the illness, or what has happened?
- What personal resources does the patient have?
- Have I got sufficient time to spend with the patient?
- Can someone else look after my bleep for an hour?
- Are there any 'what if . . .' questions I should prepare myself for? (e.g. 'What if he discharges himself?'; 'What if she gets angry with me?')

Pause, think and pre-empt difficulties before seeing the patient. In giving bad news, more difficulties arise from not thinking clearly about what you are doing and how best to achieve it than from not having answers to some of the patient's questions.

The physical setting

The ideal setting is a private room that is reasonably comfortable, free from interruptions, and has a calm ambience. Of course, such a setting is not always possible, and bad news is often given in open wards, semi-private rooms, casualty departments and patients' homes. In these settings, some attempt should be made to ensure privacy and comfort. A curtain should be drawn around a patient on an open ward if it is not possible to move to a private room. A 'do not disturb' sign should be posted on the door of the room used by others in a busy setting, such as a casualty department.

Your physical position in relation to the patient is important. Being seated conveys that you intend to stay and that the meeting will not be rushed. If the patient is in bed, it is more difficult to maintain the same eye level. It is a matter of personal choice where one sits. Some doctors prefer to sit on the side of the bed, but this can feel intrusive and too close for the patient. Sitting on an office chair beside the bed is preferable to lounging back in a comfortable chair. Others prefer to adopt the defensive position of leaning against a wall close to the patient: this conveys a relaxed posture and a commitment to remain in the room.

There are some obvious things you should not do:

● Don't give bad news at the end of a physical examination while the patient is still undressed.
● Don't give bad news in corridors and over the telephone (if this can be avoided).
● Don't pace around, keep looking out of the window or become distracted by activities nearby.

We sometimes rely on props in difficult situations. Where possible, avoid fumbling through clinical notes or fixing drips while talking to the patient. It is important to maintain eye contact. Undo your jacket or hang up your white coat, if you prefer: this creates a more personal and friendly ambience and also punctuates the uniqueness of the situation. It is preferable not to wear a stethoscope around your neck or have your bleep in view. Potential sources of distraction (telephone, television and radio) should be avoided.

Talking to the patient and responding to concerns

Whatever you tell the patient, it is essential that you do it slowly, or at least at the pace dictated by the patient. Conversation usually becomes more formal and embroidered when giving bad news. Monosyllabic replies are avoided. It would be unusual to reply with an emphatic 'no' to a relative and walk away on being asked if a patient had survived an operation. Instead, one might say:

> "As you know, your uncle was very unwell before the operation. We did the best we could, but I'm afraid that was not enough. He never regained consciousness, and I'm sorry to tell you he died shortly after the operation."

Complex information should be delivered with the minimum of medical jargon and the doctor should be empathic to the patient's needs and concerns. Failure to attend to these points may render the encounter ineffective, unhelpful or destructive to the patient. Breaking bad news requires:

- empathy
- starting with what the patient or relative already knows or understands
- finding out what the patient wants to know
- active listening, giving information, inviting feedback and addressing concerns
- eliciting the patient's own resources for coping
- instilling realistic hope.

Empathy

It should not be too difficult to empathise with someone who has suffered loss or been give bad news as most of us can readily identify with someone who faces or experiences adversity. As we saw earlier in Chapter 2 in the section on empathy, being able to put yourself in the place of another person, particularly someone who may be distressed, helps us to communicate with that individual more compassionately and effectively. Whilst some people can more easily communicate with patients about highly sensitive and potentially emotive topics, everyone can benefit from acquiring or enhancing their skills in this area. Empathy is conveyed in two different ways. Listening attentively to patients and attempting to understand their predicament more fully is one description of empathy. You are also being empathic by not introducing new information too quickly, and not imposing views and making assumptions. For example:

DR FRYER:	*The results suggest that it's not just an 'ordinary' lump.*
MRS BLACK:	*This sounds like bad news.*
DR FRYER:	*I was hoping to be able to reassure you. It seems that some of the cells we looked at were abnormal. It is important, though, that we picked this up early.*
MRS BLACK:	*Are you saying it's the big 'C'?*
DR FRYER:	*Yes, it probably is cancer.*
MRS BLACK:	*We all know what that means . . . .*
DR FRYER:	*I realise this probably comes as a shock to you.*

Warmth and caring should be conveyed to the patient. The way in which you introduce the topic of bad news will influence, to some degree, how the patient responds. It is sometimes helpful to embroider a little and use prefaces such as: 'I was wondering whether you had ever thought what it would mean if this infection does not clear up as quickly as last time?' Putting yourself down also encourages the patient to talk more freely. For example: 'You may think that some of my questions are a bit odd, but I can't help wondering whether . . .'. Showing patients that you are not afraid to discuss their concerns, no matter what these may be, is a way of showing empathy.

Start with what the patient already knows

Before giving bad news, it is useful to have an up-to-date impression of what the patient understands and believes about the illness. This will directly affect how you give the news. A patient who is overly optimistic or who does not apparently understand the serious implications of the illness will need to be introduced to the news more gradually. There are a number of questions that can be asked in order to find out what the patient already knows and may be expecting. For example:

"Did Dr Smith discuss with you what he had in mind in sending you to this clinic?"

"How have things been for you? What do you make of that?"

"Have you had any thoughts about what this may be?"

"What first went through your mind when you found the lump?"

In order to discern the patient's understanding of the prognosis (and, therefore, the seriousness of the situation), you could also ask:

"Do you know anyone else who has had a similar problem? What has happened to them?"

"Do you know about any of the treatments that can be used for this?"

"How worried are you about this?"

In some cases, patients may give the impression of knowing very little about their condition despite previous consultations. They may either be hoping that new information has come to light that contradicts previous hints of bad news, or they may not want to hear bad news. These both indicate denial of the severity of the illness, and it may be necessary first to remind the patient of the previous conversations in a non-confrontational manner. Similarly, you should pay close attention to the patient's responses to questions, emotional state and intellectual level, as these directly affect what may need to be explained in more detail, and how best to do this. It is important to check patients' understanding of certain terms. Some patients, for example, may think that a tumour means they don't have cancer, or they may mistakenly assume that common symptoms, such as nausea and weight loss, can be treated and cured as successfully as if they did not have cancer.

Find out what the patient wants to know

Having established what the patient already knows, you can begin to update the patient's knowledge and understanding. However, because you may not be clear about what the patient wants to be told, and at what stage, you first need to find out by asking: 'What would you like to be told? Is there anything you would prefer not to hear about?' Once the rules for communication are established, you are free from having to make difficult judgements about what to say. You thus avoid being blamed, or feeling embarrassed. The patient feels a sense of control over his or her management. Problems that later present in the doctor–patient relationship may be traced back to a lack of clarity about what the patient wanted to be told. The following questions help to open up conversation on this important issue:

> *"It is helpful to us to hear from you what you want to be told about your condition. Is there anything you would prefer not to be told?"*

> *"What would you like to be told about the diagnosis?"*

> *"How will we know from you what you want to be told?"*

> *"Do you want to know all the details about the diagnosis, tests and treatments, or do you just want to have an outline of what is going on?"*

> *"You say you only want to be told when there is 'good news'. What should we do if we have bad news?"*

Active listening, giving information, inviting feedback and addressing concerns

First establish rapport and trust. Active listening involves responding to questions and concerns while at the same time leading the conversation. This can be facilitated by the use of questions in conversation. For example:

> DR WATTS: *Now, is there anything you would like to ask me?*
>
> MRS PARKER: *What happens if the treatment is unsuccessful?*
>
> DR WATTS: *In many cases, the symptoms come back. We can control symptoms such as nausea and pain with certain drugs. Do you have any other concerns?*
>
> MRS PARKER: *I don't know what to say to my children – or to my mother.*
>
> DR WATTS: *This is all very recent news and perhaps you have not yet had enough time to think about how to tell others. Is there anyone else's opinions and advice you would value in deciding how to deal with your children and mother?*
>
> MRS PARKER: *My sister. She's the one we all turn to at difficult times.*

One advantage of eliciting the patient's concerns at an early stage is that problems and practical issues can be attended to, thereby reducing anxiety. Patients can also be helped to plan ahead of crises and to think in advance about problems and how they might cope with them. On the other hand, some patients may not want to look to the future, feeling that such a conversation might tempt fate. Others might become unsettled, so they should not be pushed into a discussion about their future.

Information should be given incrementally. Start with known facts, add to them, and conclude with an opinion of what all the information may mean. Once the patient has understood these details, introduce options for treatment and care. For example:

> DR MILLER: *If you remember, after you told us about the numbness in your legs and dizziness, we carried out some neurological tests. When we examined you, you also said you were having some*

> *difficulties with your vision. I mentioned to you earlier on that one of the possibilities we have to consider is multiple sclerosis. At this stage, I would like to carry out some further tests.*

MR FRANKS: *But there's no cure for MS.*

DR MILLER: *I'm afraid that's right. But there are certain treatments and new drugs that are being tried out.*

Remember that helping a patient understand the implications of bad news is not a psychotherapy session. However, it is important at least to elicit their feelings and address concerns. For example:

DR SEEDAT: *What is your main concern now that I have told you what may happen?*

MR THOMAS: *Being in pain. And not being able to look after myself.*

DR SEEDAT: *I can understand your concerns. I'd like to discuss both of them with you.*

Elicit the patient's resources for coping, and instil realistic hope

You should discuss how the patient has previously coped with personal difficulties. This helps make explicit what resources the individual has and what additional support the patient may need. The patient's natural support network should also be identified. Here are some examples of questions:

"Have you ever been given news in the past that made you feel frightened and unsure how to respond?"

"How did you deal with it?"

"How might this experience help you in what we have been discussing today?"

Information about treatments may enable patients to consider other possible outcomes of their illness. This helps to convey some hope for the future, as shown in the following example:

DR BECK: *These drugs should help to reduce the size of the lump. That should mean that you will probably have full use of your arm again. The other infections will probably have to be treated differently. What do you know about treatments for cancer?*

MRS DAVIS: *Chemotherapy. But that makes your hair fall out, doesn't it?*

DR BECK: *Yes, there are some unpleasant side-effects. I'm not sure that we need to consider that at this stage. We should first see whether a series of injections will help.*

MRS DAVIS: *Will I be cured or do I have to be treated for life?*

DR BECK: *We hope that things will get better after this course of treatment. You may find that the treatment is unpleasant. I can't say whether you'll be cured. We will need to keep a close eye on things and repeat this course of treatment.*

Arranging for follow-up or referral

After a patient has been given bad news, the last few moments of the meeting are particularly important, as the patient's main concerns inevitably arise now if they have not already been addressed. It is tempting to assume that patients have retained and understood what they have been told. Asking patients to summarise what they remember is a way to check what they have retained. If you do not correct any misunderstandings now, patients may recall only the positive or negative aspects of the news, both of which may increase the risk of reactive depression, denial, anxiety and even suicide. A plan should be made for follow-up contact to contain some of their anxiety and provide a further opportunity to address concerns. In some cases it may be appropriate to make a referral to another professional, such as a psychologist or counsellor, for specialist help with bereavement, anxiety and depression, and personal and relationship difficulties.

Feedback and handover to colleagues

It is good practice to inform colleagues about the meeting with the patient, summarise what the patient, and others, have been told and understand, and what possible problems or reactions can be expected. This helps others caring for the patient to know what to say without confusing or upsetting the patient with different information about prognosis and treatment. Discussion and consultation with colleagues can also make the task of giving bad news easier by increasing professional support and exploring ideas about how else the patient could have been managed.

Case example 5.1 *Breaking the news of breast cancer*	Mrs Ball (46 years old) had a malignant growth surgically removed from her breast after several weeks of worrying about the lump. She had felt too frightened to tell her husband or doctor but eventually went to her GP when she started to lose weight and had difficulty sleeping. After being told the results of various tests, she was seen together with her husband. This case illustrates the important skills in delivering bad news, even when there is uncertainty as to the prognosis: convey sympathy; be practical; be circumspect; and display an openness about the prognosis and the patient's views on management.

> MRS BALL: *It's all my fault. If I'd come earlier, it wouldn't have turned out this way.*
>
> DR DAY: *It seems unlikely that you could have done anything to change what has happened. The fact that you came so that we could operate on you and treat you is important.*
>
> MR BALL: *My wife always blames herself. If only she had told me earlier. It really upsets me that you worried about this all on your own. Will she get better, doctor?*

DR DAY:	From the tests we have carried out, we're confident that we are able to remove all of the tumour from the breast. We will need to find out now if it has spread to anywhere else. If it has, it will depend on where it has spread to and what damage it has already caused. How worried are you both about this?
MRS BALL:	I'm a pessimist. My husband is the eternal optimist. I know that when you start to lose weight, that's a bad sign.
DR DAY:	Mr Ball?
MR BALL:	I feel I have to be optimistic, but this time I'm very worried.
DR DAY:	What is your main worry?
MR BALL:	That I'll lose my wife (cries, the couple embrace).
DR DAY:	It is not easy saying this, but there is a chance that your wife may not get any better. Are there any immediate decisions or problems facing you?
MRS BALL (CRYING):	I was going to start working again in the next few months and one of the children is going to university later on this year.
DR DAY:	How do you see your illness affecting these?
MRS BALL:	We'll have to put everything on hold until we know where all this is going to. But I don't want my daughter staying home to look after me.
DR DAY:	Have you thought about how you are going to tell your children?
MR BALL:	We will be completely open with them both. If things don't improve, can we still expect my wife to come home soon?
DR DAY:	I can't see why not. It is important to keep an open mind about decisions until we have more information from the tests and investigations. I cannot yet be certain as to what the outlook is. We will try to arrange for your wife to leave hospital towards the end of the week. I realise it must be stressful for you both not yet having a clear idea of how things will turn out. You can help me by telling me what you would like to know about the results.
MRS BALL:	You can tell us everything. But I would prefer it if my husband were here with me when you have the results.
DR DAY:	We will certainly try to arrange for you to be seen together.

'What to do if...'

Medical students and doctors often ask: 'What do I do if a patient cries, or becomes angry, or threatens suicide?' Although these reactions are common, it is nearly impossible to predict how a patient will react to bad news, even if the patient is well known to us. It is important, however, to act in a supportive and professional manner. Whatever advice may be appropriate to the specific situation, only act in a way that is congruent with your own feelings and within the limits of professional conduct. For example, if you are uncomfortable holding a patient's hand while he cries, do not do so; it will probably come across as contrived and awkward.

What if the patient cries?

Usually, you would give the patient some tissues, or pause, or say: 'I can see you are very upset'. Although some doctors advocate touching (for example, on the shoulder or arm), be careful not to seem intrusive. It is usually inappropriate, for example, to hug or kiss a patient. After a few moments, you should continue talking, even if the patient is still crying. Very few patients will object, or feel offended, provided the doctor remains sympathetic. For example: 'I am sorry to have to give you this news. It's not easy for me. Were you expecting to hear this?' By way of contrast, it would be inappropriate to say 'Cheer up. Things could be worse'.

STOP AND THINK *How would you react if a close friend shared some recent bad news with you and started to cry? What do you think the friend might expect of you? How would you know what to do?*

What if the patient becomes angry or violent?

STOP AND THINK *Think about a situation – such as someone trying to take your parking space – and you get into an argument. What is likely to inflame the situation and possibly lead to violence?*

If confronted by an angry patient, you should stand up. The patient will usually have already stood up, and it is important to be at the patient's eye level, and to show your preparedness. You should be polite and firm. The threat of violence should always be taken seriously, and the occasion of giving bad news is no exception. In an apologetic, but firm tone, you might say: 'I'm sorry to have to give you this news. I realise that you weren't expecting to hear this. However, you may also want to speak to someone else and get their opinion'. It is sometimes helpful to add: 'I can see that you are upset and annoyed. I would be happy to try and answer any of your questions'. As a last resort, if you fear for your safety, open the door or leave the room. Having a colleague nearby may diffuse the situation.

If the patient threatens suicide

In most cases, patients can be talked out of harming themselves or resorting to suicide. However, this demands patience, care and reassurance. If the patient hints at suicide, make your concerns explicit. For example: 'I was wondering where you're going from here?' Open discussion about suicidal feelings can be containing for the patient and conveys that you are not afraid to confront sensitive issues. A patient who hints at or who threatens suicide should not be discharged or left alone.

The opinion of a psychiatrist or psychologist must be sought in cases where the patient remains suicidal.

Telling parents they have an abnormal baby

Pregnancy and childbirth are emotional experiences, and to this can be added the fear of parents that their baby might die or be born with a disability. Nearly 1 in 40 babies are born with a handicap or abnormality. The following events are associated with having to give bad news to the parents and family:

- fetus dies during pregnancy or labour
- fetus has a detectable abnormality, for which a termination may be indicated
- fetus has a detectable abnormality not requiring termination
- an abnormality is detected only after the baby is born
- a congenital condition becomes detectable in the infant's first weeks or months of life.

Tests and scans make it easier to diagnose many conditions at an early stage, and for this reason parents expect to learn of problems much earlier on in the pregnancy. The following guidelines can be followed when telling parents that their child has an abnormality:

1. Parents should be told of the problems as soon as possible. They should preferably be told together. A single mother should be asked if she would like someone with her, such as a parent, or close friend or relative. Parents often have hints that all is not well from the facial expressions of those caring for them. Telling them early on helps them to adjust to the bad news, before they have to face telling excited and hopeful friends and relatives.

2. The most senior person should break the news to them. A consultant paediatrician may need to work closely with the obstetrician in planning how to do this.

3. It may be helpful to make a drawing of the abnormality. Say, for example: 'It looks something like this, but not as large.' The explanation should be brief and simple. Those characteristics or features should be pointed out that lead one to think that it is an abnormality. Avoid giving too much detail at this stage.

4. Parents are often afraid of what they will see. Encourage them first to hold the baby. The baby should be wrapped in a blanket with only its face showing. This allows the couple to be gradually introduced to the baby and the abnormality. The couple should also be persuaded to name the baby, and the name should be used by the doctor and colleagues. For example: 'Little Ewan has a strong grip', or 'Hannah has a lovely smile'.

5. Positive features should be emphasised, although a balanced and realistic view should be presented. For example: 'He seems very healthy, though you will probably find that because of the problem

with his lip it is difficult to breast-feed him. We will need to give you some advice about this'.

6. The parents often have a mixed response to the child. On the one hand, they want to cuddle, nurture and protect the baby. On the other hand, they may feel bereaved, and experience feelings of guilt, sadness and loss, or they may be inclined to reject the child. Firstly, the parents should be reassured that this is a normal reaction. Secondly, they should not feel responsible for the abnormality.

7. Some parents may not believe what they are being told and may ignore or dismiss problems. A failure to thrive and the loss of developmental milestones may become evident in the future (such as with some children born with HIV infection), and parents should be given follow-up appointments so that the child can be monitored at regular intervals.

8. Counselling can help parents to overcome their embarrassment and reluctance to inform relatives and friends. It can also help them bond with the baby where they may have ambivalent feelings towards it.

9. When parents and baby leave hospital, they lose a supportive environment. Many new problems may only become obvious at this time. Parents should be given details of organisations that can provide further information and support.

10. If the baby has died, there are practical considerations (such as suppression of lactation for the mother and making arrangements for the funeral). The parents should have the opportunity to say goodbye to the baby, and they may want to hold and cuddle it in the privacy of a quiet room. Some parents want to keep a memento, such as a lock of hair or a blanket.

11. As in clinical situations where bad news must be given, it is important to ensure that the feelings of professional colleagues (e.g. midwives, health visitors) are attended to through discussion and support.

Key points

- Giving bad news is among the most challenging of tasks in medical practice.
- The way bad news is given affects how people cope and adjust.
- Keep an open mind as to what is 'bad news'. Some patients are distressed by seemingly good news, whereas others experience some relief on hearing bad news.
- Before giving bad news, consider to whom it should be given, who should give it, when it should be given and what are the likely consequences of giving it.
- It helps to find out what the patient already knows and may want to be told. Making assumptions about either of these can lead to serious problems in management.

- Giving bad news requires time, a setting free from distractions or interruptions, empathy, active listening and humility to say that you may not have the answers to certain questions.
- Elicit the patient's own resources for coping and instil realistic hope.
- Ensure that colleagues know what the patient has been told.
- Provide support for the patient's relatives and your professional colleagues.

FURTHER READING

Barnett M 2002 Effect of breaking bad news on patients' perceptions of doctors. Journal of the Royal Society of Medicine 95: 343–347

Buckman R 1992 How to break bad news. Papermac, London

Fallowfield L, Jenkins V 2004 Communicating bad, sad and difficult news in medicine. Lancet 363: 312–319

Leff P, Walizer E 1992 The uncommon wisdom of parents at the moment of diagnosis. Family Systems Medicine 10: 147–168

Ptacek J, Ellison N 2001 I'm sorry to tell you...Physicians' reports of breaking bad news. Journal of Behavioural Medicine 24: 205–217

Simpson R, Bor R 2001 I'm not picking up a heartbeat. Experience of sonographers giving bad news to women during ultrasound. British Journal of Medical Psychology 74: 255–272

6

Taking a sexual history

Why is it important to talk about sex?

Special skills are required for soliciting a sexual history from a patient. Although it may seem easier to communicate with patients about their sexual problems in a genitourinary medicine clinic, medical and social problems, such as sexual dysfunction, sexually transmitted infections and especially HIV and hepatitis C, confront us in most clinical settings with complex and sensitive issues that have to be raised with our patients. In many instances patients go to the doctor to discuss sexual problems, but during the consultation become inhibited and fail to raise their concerns. Patients sometimes worry that they will feel judged or ridiculed. Doctors and medical students working in a wide range of settings need to acquire some basic skills that enable them to take a sexual history. These skills convey to the patient that the clinician is not embarrassed to talk about sexual problems, whether these are the reason for seeking medical care or stem from another medical problem.

There are seven main reasons why medical students and doctors experience difficulty talking to patients about sex:

1. There may be embarrassment and personal unease with the subject.
2. Medical students may feel that they are too young to ask older patients details about their sexual relationships.
3. The student or doctor may be concerned that the patient may feel offended.
4. There could be a belief that a sexual history is not relevant to the complaint.
5. It may be assumed that this should be someone else's task, e.g. a specialist in genitourinary medicine or a sexual health adviser.
6. There may be a lack of skills in dealing with complex problems, such as the patient's personal relationships and problems stemming from the patient keeping secrets.
7. The student may feel inadequately trained for the task.

Table 6.1 Common assumptions and misconceptions about sexuality
• Elderly people don't have sex

- Elderly people don't have sex
- Gay men only have sex with men
- A married person couldn't possibly have a sexually transmitted disease (STD)
- Patients with sexual problems will recognise them and attend an STD clinic
- Young people under the legal age don't have sex
- Everyone understands the basics of reproduction
- Patients will raise the issue of sexual problems with their doctor if they have any concerns
- The presence of sexual problems usually means that the patient also has psychological problems
- All patients understand medical terms doctors tend to use when describing sexual activities and the genitalia
- You can tell a person's sexual orientation by his or her appearance

Further barriers to open communication about sexual problems in a clinical setting include stereotypes and unchallenged assumptions about people's lifestyle and behaviour (Table 6.1). Assumptions such as gay men never have sex with women and the elderly do not have sexual relations are both incorrect and may prevent history-taking and counselling about important issues.

Gender differences and cultural rules may further complicate the doctor–patient relationship where sexual problems need to be discussed. Some female patients may feel uncomfortable discussing intimate issues with a male doctor or medical student (and vice versa). They may dismiss any suggestion of a sexual problem, fearing that the doctor or medical student would want to examine them. Most patients feel both vulnerable and self-conscious being physically examined, and these feelings are more intense where the genitalia are the main focus of the examination.

Our personal attitudes towards sexual practices and lifestyle may influence how sexual problems are discussed with patients. We convey to patients (through verbal and non-verbal communication) indifference, acceptance or rejection of sexual practices and lifestyles. The subtle hints we give about personal values and views about lifestyle will influence patients in deciding whether to keep important information secret and go elsewhere for their care.

When to talk about sex

Conversations about sex and soliciting a detailed sex history may be required in the following situations.

Where patients present with a problem that is likely to be sexually related

Symptoms such as a genital discharge would normally lead to a discussion with the doctor about past sexual activities, a physical examination, counselling about reducing further risk to the patient and other sexual partners and treatment. A patient's anxiety about sexual performance might also present to the doctor in this context.

When patients have medical or social problems that may lead to sexual difficulties

Sexual problems may be associated with other medical or social problems. Impotence resulting from diabetes and infertility are examples of these, as is a person with HIV worrying about disclosure of this status to a partner when starting a new relationship.

When sexual problems are not related to medical treatment

Problems concerning sexual matters not directly related to medical treatment may have implications for patient care. Sexual relationships in hospital, both between patients and between patients and their visitors (including spouses), are forbidden. Problems arising from lack of sexual intimacy in relationships among hospitalised patients may need to be addressed with patients. On wards and in units where patients have a diminished ability to make rational and informed decisions, more complex questions are raised. Finally, sexual harassment of staff (usually female doctors and nurses) by either patients or colleagues has implications for professionalism and relationships, apart from the obvious legal ramifications, and may need to be discussed openly.

Should a sexual history be solicited from all patients?

Medical problems frequently have implications for a person's relationships and sexual functioning. Psychological problems may mask concerns about sex, sexual functioning and sexual health. It is also possible that some psychological problems, including depression, anxiety, insomnia and phobias, may be symptoms of underlying sexual problems.

The questions a doctor chooses to ask when taking a medical history imply clinical decision-making. The interview proceeds according to the patient's problem and mental state and the doctor's knowledge and experience of medical problems. It is clear that where a patient complains of a problem that is obviously of a sexual nature, it is necessary to take a sexual history. By way of contrast, some sexual problems are either masked by, or the result of, a related problem. In these circumstances, there may be a dilemma as to whether it is appropriate or timely to take a sexual history from the patient. The advantages and disadvantages of taking a sexual history in these circumstances are set out in Table 6.2.

Table 6.2 Advantages and difficulties of taking a routine sexual history

Advantages	Difficulties
• Sexual problems are seen as a normal part of the spectrum of problems discussed with a doctor • By talking about sexual issues, even when they are not seen as problems, you open the door for future consultations about sexual problems • Discussion about sexual activities can be an opportunity for health promotion	• It may be embarrassing for the patient and doctor • The patient may misinterpret the purpose of the discussion and feel that his or her lifestyle is being judged or condemned • The patient may begin to worry about something that was not previously a problem

There is a difference between asking a patient in the course of taking a medical history whether he or she has any sexual or relationship problems, and taking a detailed sexual history. Since HIV became a major medical and social problem in the early 1980s, it has become important to raise the matter of sexual health with a wide range of patients. Hepatitis C is likely to become a focal point for testing and treatment in the context of sexual health in the coming years. There are guidelines for obtaining informed consent before taking blood tests, carrying out laboratory tests, investigations and starting treatment. The starting point for determining whether a more extensive sexual history should be taken from a patient who does not voluntarily raise concerns about sexual health could be to ask if the patient has any questions about sexual health or, specifically, about HIV, in the light of media publicity. In so doing, we acknowledge the need to provide health education to all patients without having to make assumptions about their lifestyle or personal relationships.

Guidelines for talking about sex (Fig. 6.1)

(p. 192)   **Exercise 7**   The following guidelines offer hints as to how to talk to patients about issues relating to sex. Using questions during the interview will help you to guard against lecturing, or making assumptions about lifestyle and sexual relationships.

The setting

The setting in which interviews take place directly influences what can be achieved. An open ward, which offers little privacy to the patient, a genitourinary medicine clinic, a gynaecology ward, consulting rooms

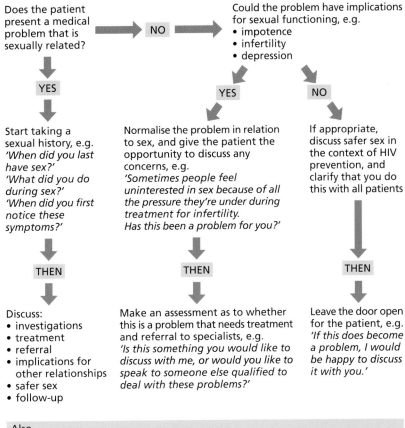

Fig. 6.1 Algorithm for deciding when and how to take a sexual history.

in a GP practice and a nurses' station on a ward are different settings in which sexual matters are sometimes raised.

You should ensure that the setting is appropriate for taking a sexual history and that there is privacy so that the conversation can be seen to be confidential. A second consideration is whether the doctor feels comfortable discussing sexual matters with patients. If you feel uncomfortable, you might prefer to identify the patient's problem and then suggest that the patient is interviewed by someone on the staff with greater experience. Finally, there are considerations of personal safety. In some circumstances, it may be preferable for more than one person to be present during the conversation, particularly if there is the suspicion that the patient might become violent or abusive. Although this may compromise privacy, safety should be a primary consideration.

Introductions

After introducing yourself, a handshake or touch can communicate to the patient that he or she is not 'dirty' or 'bad'. The confidential nature of the session should be stressed.

Start with the presenting problem

The discussion should start with the presenting problem and progress to more sensitive areas. Some patients may need prompting or encouragement to talk about sexual problems. They should be given the opportunity to raise more sensitive issues. At the end of a discussion about other problems, you might ask a general question, such as:

"Is there anything else you would like to discuss with me?"

"I'm not sure that I have given you the opportunity to talk about everything you had in mind to discuss in coming to see me. Is there perhaps something about a relationship or a sexual matter that you wanted to talk about?"

Be purposeful

Where it is important for the doctor to open the discussion and solicit information, it is helpful to be purposeful and direct. For example:

"I need to find out something about your relationships to help make an assessment of this problem. I would like to ask you some personal questions about your sexual relationships."

You might add to this:

"People sometimes feel a bit embarrassed about these questions. I just wanted you to know that I am perfectly comfortable discussing these sort of issues."

Gather further information to provide a comprehensive sexual history

Addressing the presenting problem is but one aspect of history-taking. There may also be a need to gather a more comprehensive history. This could include information about some of the following:

- age of first sexual experience
- nature of previous sexual activities
- history of pregnancies, miscarriages, contraceptive or barrier protection methods used
- history of other sexually transmitted diseases, relevant factors, such as travel away from home, alcohol and drug use
- history of sexual abuse

- psychological problems
- psychosexual problems (erection, ejaculation, loss of sexual desire, pain during intercourse)
- cultural and religious rules and practices.

Remain non-judgemental about lifestyle

Initial embarrassment about describing sexual activities can be offset if preceded by an assessment of relationships. You should ask neutral questions that do not presume the gender of a partner or the nature of the patient's relationships:

"Do you have a regular partner?"

"How many other partners have you had?"

"When did you last have a sexual contact?"

Assumptions should not be made as to whether these relationships are with people of the same sex, opposite sex or both. In order to determine the nature of the activities, you should avoid asking the patient: 'Are you gay?', 'Are you heterosexual?', 'Are you promiscuous?', or 'Are you unfaithful?' Questions such as these may lead to stereotyping and cause offence. As a rule, we find that questions about activities are more useful than questions about lifestyle or sexual orientation. One might ask:

"Was this with a man or a woman, or both?"

"Have you previously had a sexual relationship with a man or woman?"

The implications of a sexual problem for the patient's personal relationships should also be addressed:

"So your wife does not know you have this discharge today from your penis. But you say you had intercourse with her last week. What might happen if we treat you and then she has symptoms of infection, such as a discharge? What might you say to her?"

Remain non-judgemental about sexual activities

The specific nature of sexual activities will need to be clarified in the course of history-taking. The doctor should encourage the patient to elaborate on a statement such as: 'We had sex together'. It sometimes helps to use the patient's own words in formulating questions:

MR TOBIN: *We got into bed together.*
DR ROSE: *Can you tell me what happened between you when you were in bed together?*
MR TOBIN: *We had sex.*
DR ROSE: *When you had sex together, was this vaginal sex, anal sex or both?*

Patients may feel embarrassed to describe a particular sexual activity. By discussing a list of sexual activities, the embarrassment or mystique surrounding the naming of activities disappears. This paves the way for the patient to be more open about discussing sexual activities:

> "You say you had sex. Can I check with you, does that mean you touched each other? Had oral sex? Masturbated one another? Had penetrative sex?"

Assumptions should not be made about terms that are not understood. For example, a doctor might have to ask:

> "I don't think I understand what you mean by 'rimming'. Can you please explain to me what it means?"

It is also important to remain neutral and not ascribe personal notions of normality or abnormality to sexual activities. Reactions of shock or surprise should be avoided. Questions about sexual experience should be framed in a positive way. It is better to ask: 'When did you last have sex?' than 'Have you ever had sex?', because a more honest answer is likely to be forthcoming.

It is advisable to use simple words rather than medical terminology. On the other hand, colloquial or 'street language' may be offensive and compromise professionalism. First check the patient understands terminology for sexual activities or parts of the anatomy, as some seemingly obvious terms may be misunderstood.

Use the opportunity for health education

Patients' concerns about sexual and other medical problems are opportunities for general health education. In order to be meaningful and appropriate to the patient, promoting healthy lifestyle and behaviours should take into account the age and developmental stage of the patient, as well as cultural and religious factors:

> DR GOLDIN: Now that you have heard that you have a negative HIV antibody test result, what might help you to keep the result that way?
>
> MR PAYE: Sleeping around less.
>
> DR GOLDIN: Yes, but it's also important that you think about what you do during sex that is risky. What about using condoms when you have sex?

Refer to appropriate specialists

A range of professionals may need to be called on to assess patients with sexually related problems, including physicians in genitourinary medicine, health advisers, surgeons, urologists, gynaecologists, marriage and sex therapists, counsellors, psychologists and psychiatrists.

Case example 6.1

A married man worried he might have contracted HIV

Mr Jones, aged 32, came to the accident and emergency department one evening and was clerked by a fifth-year medical student. He was worried that he had AIDS because he had had an affair with a woman while on a business trip 3 years ago. The student began by asking why he had become worried at this point. Note how the student uses neutral terms until the point where the patient makes clear the nature of his relationships and sexual activities:

MR JONES: *I've had night sweats and diarrhoea.*

STUDENT: *For how long?*

MR JONES: *A week.*

STUDENT: *Have you had a test for HIV before, or investigations for any other sexually transmitted diseases?*

MR JONES: *No.*

STUDENT: *Do you have any other symptoms at the moment?*

MR JONES: *I can't sleep I'm so worried.*

STUDENT: *First we will need to examine you, and then we can talk about the different tests we can do. A qualified doctor will join us in a short while. In the meantime, I'd like to ask you a few more questions. Are you in a relationship with anyone?*

MR JONES: *I'm married. My wife doesn't know I'm here. She doesn't know anything about what I got up to.*

STUDENT: *Do you and your wife have a sexual relationship?*

MR JONES: *Of sorts. It hasn't been very good since we had our last child 4 years ago. There's never been anyone else except the prostitute overseas.*

STUDENT: *I need to check with you whether you have sex with your wife.*

MR JONES: *Occasionally.*

STUDENT: *Do you use any form of contraception?*

MR JONES: *She's on the pill and we also use condoms. She finds sex a bit messy!*

STUDENT: *Is there any other way in which anything could be passed on to her during sex?*

MR JONES: *I don't think so; she doesn't like oral sex.*

STUDENT: *What sort of sex did you have with the prostitute?*

MR JONES: *Intercourse. We used a condom. But I can't remember if it broke. I'd been drinking.*

STUDENT: *Was this anal or vaginal intercourse?*

MR JONES: *No, just 'straight'.*

STUDENT: *Did you notice any symptoms in the few days after you had intercourse; maybe a discharge from your penis, any sores, itching?*

MR JONES: *Not that I remember. There's nothing like that now, anyway. What's the risk of AIDS if you use a condom?*

STUDENT: *Condoms certainly reduce the risk of becoming infected, if used properly. There may be a small risk of infection when condoms tear or slip off. The biggest risk is having anal or vaginal intercourse with someone who is infected and not using a condom. The problem is that it's very difficult to tell whether you are infected unless you have been tested, or you are very unwell. Ah, here's Dr Smith.*

The medical student handed over to the doctor and summarised the main points of the discussion. The patient was examined and given an appointment for the following day at the genitourinary medicine clinic. It was explained to him that he would be examined and tested for a number of infections. He would also receive counselling before he made a final decision to be tested for HIV so that he was informed of the implications of the test and result. The patient returned to the accident and emergency department a week later to tell the staff that no sexually transmitted diseases had been diagnosed, his HIV test result was negative and his sleep pattern had improved. He had also been given a leaflet describing safer sex activities.

Case example 6.2

Treating a man who was depressed and presented with impotence

The last patient to be seen at the GP surgery was Mr Keys, a 40-year-old engineer. Dr Whincup introduced the patient to Theresa, a medical student who was on placement to the practice. Mr Keys looked apprehensive and said that he would prefer to be seen without the student being present. Dr Whincup explained that it was important for the student to learn about different problems, but would respect his views. As the student got up to leave, Mr Keys said that he wouldn't mind after all if she remained in the room. The consultation began with the patient saying:

MR KEYS: *You see it's all rather personal and embarrassing.*

DR WHINCUP: *Perhaps I should assure you that even though I have a student here, our discussion is all in the strictest confidence. Can you say a bit more about why this may be embarrassing?*

MR KEYS: *It's about sex. Things just aren't the same.*

DR WHINCUP: *How long have things been different?*

MR KEYS: *About a month.*

DR WHINCUP: *What has most changed for you?*

MR KEYS: *I don't know how else to say it, but I simply don't enjoy it like I used to.*

DR WHINCUP: *What did you used to enjoy doing?*

MR KEYS: *Sex with my wife. Now I can't do it.*

DR WHINCUP: *Can't do it?*

MR KEYS: *Get an erection. I feel very foolish saying this to you. And it makes me feel awful about my wife.*

DR WHINCUP: *Is this something that you have discussed with her?*

MR KEYS: *Not really. I try to avoid having sex.*

DR WHINCUP: *You don't have any sex at all at the moment?*

MR KEYS: *I see what you're getting at! No, none.*

DR WHINCUP:	*Just a few questions: when did you last have an erection? Do you usually have an erection in the morning when you wake up?*
MR KEYS:	*Yes, usually in the morning.*
DR WHINCUP:	*That's important, and also good news. At least it means your 'equipment' isn't broken. Tell me a bit more about what's happening at home and at work.*
MR KEYS:	*My wife thinks I'm under the weather. You know – depressed. My boss is off on sick leave; he's been away for 5 weeks. My wife stopped her part-time teaching job. The kids are on holiday at the moment. And I'm not sleeping very well, and I've lost some weight.*
DR WHINCUP:	*How would you describe your mood?*
MR KEYS:	*My wife is probably right; I feel depressed.*
DR WHINCUP:	*Have you ever felt like this before?*
MR KEYS:	*I saw a psychiatrist when I was at university because I got depressed soon after I left home. He prescribed antidepressants. I don't know if they worked, or if I got better just from speaking to the psychiatrist.*
DR WHINCUP:	*It's quite common for people not to enjoy things they usually like doing when they're stressed or depressed. There may be several reasons why you are having sexual problems. The first point is that the more you put yourself under pressure to perform sexually, the less likely it is that you will spontaneously have an erection. I suspect that your body is saying to you that it's exhausted and stressed. Second, stress and sexual problems often go together. As you know, there are pills for depression, anxiety and to help with sleep. I would suggest, though, that we first look at how events in your life may be contributing to this before we talk about medication. We have a psychologist in our practice who is experienced in dealing with sexual relationships and stress-related difficulties. Would you be interested in meeting her?*
MR KEYS:	*If you think it would help.*
DR WHINCUP:	*I feel confident that it will be of some help.*

The psychologist designed a stress reduction and relaxation programme for Mr Keys. Sexual problems were dealt with using the Masters and Johnson technique, based on removing pressure on Mr Keys to feel that he had to have intercourse with his wife. The focus was shifted to the pleasures of non-penetrative sexual activities. Although he reported that he was able to get an erection during these activities, he declined the invitation to bring his wife to some sessions. His sexual performance and work-related stress showed signs of improvement. By way of contrast, his mood remained low and a course of antidepressants was prescribed by the GP. Eight weeks later, all the problems had been resolved.

Key points

- Medical and social problems, such as sexual dysfunction, sexually transmitted infections and especially HIV and hepatitis C, confront us with complex and sensitive issues that may need to be raised with patients.
- Cultural taboos, a fear of upsetting patients and lack of skills in sexual counselling are obstacles to more open communication about sexual matters in health care settings.
- There is a tendency to make assumptions about lifestyle and behaviour where stereotypic views are held.
- Sexual problems invariably have an impact on other relationships.
- Special skills can be learned that can help in counselling patients about sexual matters.
- The dos and don'ts of discussing sexual matters include:
  - be purposeful
  - don't make assumptions
  - don't stereotype
  - ask questions; don't judge people
  - use the patient's words and language
  - remain professional
  - address relationships
  - ask when you don't understand a term or activity
  - ask questions about sexual activities rather than lifestyle
  - address confidentiality and privacy.

FURTHER READING

Bor R, Gill S, Miller R et al 2008 Counselling in health care settings. Palgrave McMillan, London

Green S, Flemons D 2004 A handbook of brief sex therapy. WW Norton, New York

Merrill J, Laux L, Thornby J 1990 Why doctors have difficulty with sex histories. Southern Medical Journal 83: 613–617

Miller D, Green J 2002 The psychology of sexual health. Blackwell Science, Oxford

Vollmer S, Wells K 1988 How comfortable do first-year medical students expect to be when taking sexual histories? Medical Education 22: 418–425

7

Communicating with patients from different cultural backgrounds

Zack Eleftheriadou

The importance of cross-cultural and racial issues

Cross-cultural doctor and patient communication poses different pressures from those encountered when working with patients from the same cultural group. Patients who come from a different culture find themselves not only in a new and unfamiliar country, but also in an unfamiliar hospital environment. The hospital may represent a different set of cultural values and expectations, as well as a different language. Facing illness in a foreign environment and away from friends and family can make the whole experience extremely alienating, especially when no one speaks the patient's language.

STOP AND THINK *Imagine that you are physically unwell and don't know what is wrong. You know that you need to consult a doctor and you go to the nearest hospital. You walk into an unfamiliar building and don't know where you should go; all the signs are in another language. You hear this language being spoken and do not understand it, but you know you must make contact with someone urgently. How would you feel? What would you do? If you are already anxious about being unwell then the added pressure of the new environment can make people less able to think and less confident to manage situations effectively.*

Cross-cultural encounters are not only difficult for patients – they can make demands on the doctor, too. For example, during a medical consultation, you may have to consider racial and cultural factors unfamiliar to you, factors that can take time and patience to understand. Furthermore, you may be unsure of what are the individual's or the family's ideas and expectations and what are the cultural ideas and expectations. The following case will help us to consider the difficulties that may arise in communicating with people from different cultures.

Case example 7.1

Mrs Shah, an Asian woman attending a hospital clinic

Mrs Shah was referred to the outpatient clinic by her GP. She arrived with her husband, and the nurse called her to see the doctor. Her husband got up to go with her, but the nurse told him this was not necessary. Mr Shah was angry and insisted on talking to the doctor himself. The doctor could see that they were dressed in traditional clothes, and that their spoken English was poor. He wondered why Mr Shah was so angry and why he wanted to accompany his wife. He often felt uncomfortable dealing with patients from other cultures, as the way of relating can be so different.

The role of culture in the doctor–patient relationship

In every medical encounter you need to understand the patient's culture in order to begin to communicate effectively. Culture can be defined as ideas, values, beliefs, customs and behaviours based on different people's upbringing and personal experiences. When communicating with patients from different backgrounds, cultural differences are further highlighted by language, dress, gender issues, family relationships and attitudes to illness, amongst many other factors.[1]

The doctor may have a different cultural perspective and different concepts of health care from those of the patient. In a clinical encounter, the doctor needs to consider the patient's perspective, but this must be done without making too many assumptions based on the doctor's knowledge of the patient's background. For example, in the case example of Mrs Shah, it would be wrong to assume that she is not familiar with British culture because she is Indian and her spoken English is poor. External differences, such as dress or language, do not necessarily reflect different ideas and values. The doctor needs to find out what are the patient's expectations, ideas and beliefs without basing these ideas on the patient's appearance or language.

Before exploring the ways the doctor can begin to address cross-cultural issues, it is helpful to outline the issues that need to be addressed and explore why communication can be problematic.

STOP AND THINK *Consider the many events, procedures and routines in medical and hospital care that are likely to be new or different for the patient. Now consider which of these might especially provoke anxiety.*

When cultural issues arise in hospital, it is important that the staff feel comfortable discussing the patient's concerns and try to understand the patient's perspective. If staff are comfortable asking the questions, patients will then be made more comfortable and willing to answer, even if the questions are considered private or difficult to discuss in front of family members. It can sometimes be difficult when our own cultural practices are challenged by patients from different cultures. The text below gives examples of specific practices that could be relevant in a medical consultation. This does not imply that you need to know everything about a different culture, but you need to acknowledge the existence of different views on social practices.

Naming

- Find out the patient's full name.
- Ask if the patient has a surname different from the one usually used, as at times, patients (particularly the younger generation) may try to make their surnames more westernized so they become recognisable. However, unless clarified, this can cause a great deal of confusion.
- The names of other family members may be different, so do not use the husband's surname to refer to the wife, and vice versa. For example, in Hindi there are four different words for 'aunt' and 'uncle', and in Bengali there is no gender differentiation for common nouns and pronouns, so you may find that 'he' and 'she' are used interchangeably.
- Address people by their surnames unless a familiarity with the patient has been established. In some cultures, elders may expect to be addressed formally as a sign of respect.

Significant others

- Ask who are the significant people who have accompanied the patient to the hospital. Find out if the patient really wishes to be accompanied or feels obligated to do so.
- Find out if the significant others wish to accompany the patient during the medical interview. For example, in the case study, Mr Shah felt it was his duty, as head of the household, to be with his wife in order to explain her problem to the doctor and be directly informed about her condition. However, even if Mrs Shah is accompanied, and cultural practices are respected, it is still the duty of the doctor/nurse to make sure that she understands all the communications and procedures.
- How many people can join the patient during the medical interview and how can they be involved, and at which stage? For example, visitor restrictions and visiting hours are often difficult issues: you should clearly explain that this is hospital policy and the impact of visitors on other patients.

Food and diet

- Are there dietary rules that the patient wishes to follow? For example, a Muslim patient will not eat pork as it is considered impure.
- Is the patient vegetarian or vegan?
- Do patients have a preference about the manner in which food is served? For example, Muslim patients will not eat food offered with the left hand because only the right hand is considered to be pure and clean.

- Can relatives bring in food for the patient? If so, then clear guidance and rules have to be offered as to what is helpful for the patient's diet and recovery without offending cultural ideas on eating practices and types of food offered during sickness.

Religion

- Ask if the patient has a religion and if he or she practises it.
- Ask if the patient wishes to worship whilst in hospital, what form this might take and the frequency, and how this might be negotiated with the nursing staff on duty. Where appropriate, explore the patient's religious views that may have a bearing on procedures such as blood transfusions and abortions, for example.

Hygiene and grooming

- Are there particular wishes about bathing? For example, in Sikh culture a deceased person must be washed by someone of the same sex.
- How does the patient feel about getting undressed in front of a doctor or nurse of the opposite sex?
- Does the patient object to the shaving of the head or body?

Dress

- Are there areas of the body that have to remain covered? For example, it is vital that orthodox Muslim women keep all parts of their body covered, except for their hands.
- Do jewellery and head coverings have religious significance?
- Are there items of clothing that are particularly significant?

Who should raise cross-cultural issues?

There is some controversy as to whether the patient or the doctor should introduce issues of culture or race in the medical interview. In consequence, discussion of these issues is sometimes neglected. More recently, training in cross-cultural work has improved, and as a result professionals have taken on more responsibility to consider and initiate discussion on the significant aspects of the patient's cultural background. If cross-cultural issues are important in the encounter, they will arise at some stage, whether directly or indirectly. For example, if patients feel frustrated because their cultural needs are not taken into account, they may not comply with the treatment, or may miss appointments. This is an indirect way of letting the doctor know that something important to the patient needs to be addressed. In the case example of Mrs Shah, the doctor needs to establish:

- if it is more acceptable in her culture that she be joined by her husband rather than left alone with a male doctor
- if her hesitancy may be caused by reasons that are not related to her culture.

The doctor could invite both of them into a private room to discuss whether her husband should be present:

DOCTOR: *Would you both like to join me?*
MRS SHAH: *My husband must come with me so that he can explain to me what I have to do. I mustn't be left on my own – after all, it is my husband who has brought me here.*

In this interview, it is clear that cultural issues are present from the beginning, but if a patient hints at issues and cannot address them directly, it is the doctor's task to encourage more open discussion. If the doctor allows the issues to be expressed as part of the interview, it is less likely they will interfere in the medical process. There are several reasons why patients might sometimes present cross-cultural issues only in a covert way, or might avoid them altogether:

- They may fear that the doctor might become angry or judgemental, or will not understand the significance of the issues.
- They do not know how much the doctor knows about their culture and whether the doctor will take it seriously. They may fear that showing a preference for their own practices will insult the doctor's culture and training. They then worry that the presumed insult might interfere with their treatment.
- In some cultures, the doctor (particularly a male doctor) is a figure of very high status whose authority should not be challenged.
- Some patients may be angry at having to travel from abroad to seek treatment in an alien culture, and they may be afraid to show their anger to the doctor. As a result they may keep quiet about an aspect of the treatment, but show their uncomfortable feelings indirectly by missing appointments or non-compliance with treatment.

Why is it difficult for doctors to raise cross-cultural issues?

- Fear of sounding racist, or prejudiced about cultural issues
- Feeling inadequate and inexperienced when discussing such issues
- Not knowing enough about the culture
- Fear of misunderstanding
- Fear of rejection if suggestions are culturally unacceptable
- Uncertainty about the patient's particular background, i.e. whether the patient is an immigrant or was born into the majority culture, and which aspects of the majority culture the patient adheres to.

Barriers in cross-cultural communication (Tables 7.1 and 7.2)

Cultural values

Patients may come from cultural systems in which values, norms, beliefs and behaviours may not reflect (in reality or perceived not to reflect) those of the medical staff. Shared cultural definitions of concepts, practices and rituals help us to communicate with other groups in our society but can become barriers when we deal with people from different cultures. Cultures differ in their attitudes to family structure, marriage or partnership, child-bearing and child-rearing and, generally, in how the individual is perceived in relation to society. Some cultures place greater significance on individual identity than communal identity, whereas other cultures do the opposite. Our assumptions about other cultures can become so fixed that we expect all patients from a particular culture to think or behave in the same way. We might assume, for example, that all Bengali women must be spoken to through their husbands or another

---

Table 7.1 Advice on cross-cultural communication with patients

- Be aware of your own values so that you do not impose them on the patient
- Learn about the cultural background of your patients, particularly if they constitute a large group in your community
- Learn which cultural differences might affect treatment
- Show the patient that you respect the differences between you
- Find out if there are similarities in ideas and expectations and build on them whenever possible
- Be open-minded about cultural practices unfamiliar to you
- Accommodate cultural ideas in the treatment without compromising the quality of care provided for the patient
- Explain that you will try to give the best medical care possible, but that you are not an expert on their culture

---

Table 7.2 Dos and don'ts in cross-cultural communication

Do
- Use open questions
- Explore basic racial and cultural background issues that are considered helpful, but explore in depth only if necessary
- Be honest about anything that may be unclear to you
- Show respect for cultural differences

Don't
- Pretend to understand cultural patterns you are unclear about
- Be judgemental about cultural patterns
- Make assumptions about how the patient's cultural patterns might relate to the onset of illness or to the outcome of treatment
- Assume that cultural issues are unimportant if they don't appear in the initial interview, as they may become pertinent at any stage of the medical encounter

male relative. Although this may be true for many Bengali women, there are others who hold different views. Parents or elders may be considered the most important members of their society and should be respected. There may be clear rules regarding how different people should be addressed by the younger members. Such an attitude will inevitably enter the doctor–patient relationship, because if the patient is not used to challenging authority figures, he or she will conform with everything suggested by the doctor. The case of Mahmooda (Case example 7.2) illustrates the importance of liaising with different family members.

Another example of the importance of understanding the patient's cultural context is when working with Japanese families. For example, during a consultation the doctor is told that the patient, a 4-year-old child, is still sleeping in the parents' bedroom. The doctor's first task is to find out if this is common practice in Japan before classifying it as problematic behaviour (because it is not common practice in western societies):

"Has the child always slept in your room?"

"Is it a common practice in Japanese society for children to sleep in the parents' bedroom?"

If cultural information needs to be brought into the consultation, the doctor can ask the patient to clarify his or her cultural practices, e.g. 'Do you have arranged marriages in your family?' This way of questioning treats the patient as an individual. Individuals may have adopted some cultural ideas and rejected others, so it is misleading to assume that all their behaviour will be determined by their culture. For instance, although they share some basic ideas, the Muslim Chinese, Chinese Buddhists and the modern Chinese differ significantly in their attitude to how the body of a deceased person should be treated.

Human development

Every period of human development is defined by cultural ideas and practices. For example, in the UK, 'adolescence' refers to a particular developmental stage, identified by certain experiences, conflicts, preoccupations and goals. In another culture, adolescence may begin at a different time and have different defining characteristics. For example, it would be incorrect to assume that an Italian adolescent female is going through identical, age-related conflicts to a British girl of the same age. Because life stages differ across cultures, you need to learn about the patient's experience.

Perceptions of illness, care and treatment

Each culture has different views about acceptable and effective forms of medical treatment, health and care.[2] All patients will have some notion of how they acquired their illness and what care and treatment they need. It is helpful to try to establish what these ideas are before proceeding with the medical consultation. As the doctor, you should find out if there is common ground between their ideas and your own; otherwise the patient may feel misunderstood or frustrated because the doctor has dismissed or avoided asking about personal or cultural beliefs.

Illness can be attributed to different causes. A patient who had travelled to Europe from Africa was shocked to be diagnosed as HIV-positive because he thought it was only a 'white person's disease'. After the diagnosis, he felt that his illness was God's punishment and consequently did not see any reason for treatment if it was God's will that he should die. In this case, the doctor might find it hard to reconcile the patient's beliefs with the doctor's own knowledge. However, it is necessary to respect the patient's religious views and discuss how he can best be supported. It may be appropriate, with his consent, to find someone of his own culture who understands HIV disease and who can give him psychological support.

Language

Language is foremost among problems in cross-cultural communication. Even when the patient is familiar with the language of the majority culture, there are nuances, metaphors, idiomatic expressions and non-verbal cues that can cause misunderstanding or confusion for non-native speakers. Misunderstanding can threaten the doctor–patient relationship and also have serious implications for the patient's care.

When treating patients with little or no knowledge of English, some doctors use cards featuring key words in different languages and their English translation. The patient is shown the words of his or her own language and the doctor reads the equivalent English word. For example, the doctor can try to establish whether the patient means 'sad', 'depressed' or 'angry' by choosing the appropriate words from the pack. The card system can be used when it is difficult to find an interpreter, or to enhance communication even when an interpreter is present. Cards also enable the doctor and patient to communicate directly, rather than through a third person.

At times, published material can be useful for patients to have in their own language, but these leaflets have to be explained properly and they do not replace face-to-face medical consultations. They are often a way for patients to read further or to absorb information when they are able to think about their medical condition in a less pressurised setting.

The cultural background of the doctor

To summarise the main issues involved in working with patients from different cultural backgrounds:

- It is not necessary to raise cultural or racial issues unless they are important for the patient, or unless a misunderstanding might occur if they are not addressed.

- There is sometimes a misconception that a patient should be matched to a doctor from the same cultural or racial background in order to facilitate communication and enhance care. This may be desirable for some patients, but for others, differences in background will not be a barrier, or they may not be relevant to the treatment in any way. Patients should be able to choose whom they wish to consult and indicate how they wish to be treated. The doctor might ask, for example:

"Do you feel it would be easier to see a doctor from a similar background?"

"I can appreciate how frustrating it is to talk to someone who doesn't share your culture (or speak your native language), but perhaps you can let me know about cultural practices that are important for you to follow when you are in hospital."

The doctor acknowledges that there are communication problems and tries to work with the patient to overcome them. Alternatively, some patients may choose a doctor from a different culture, preferring not to disclose their illness to someone of their own background because they contracted it through an activity that is culturally unacceptable. For other patients, a doctor of their own gender may be more important than a doctor of their own culture. At times, matching only serves to reinforce stereotypes that groups hold about one another. Also, if a patient is matched with a doctor of the same culture, the patient may expect the doctor to share his or her values; this might place a doctor trained in a different cultural system in an awkward position.

- Patients and doctors can communicate effectively even if they are from different cultures. It is often thought that if doctor and patient are too culturally distant, they will not be able to communicate effectively. Such a belief can result in hospital staff avoiding an ethnic-minority patient because they are unsure about how to communicate. In fact, differences may not always be a barrier. You can explore ways to gain information about the patient's culture that can be used in a constructive way to complement care. It is also possible that the patient is well informed about the host country's cultural practices and is willing to look beyond his or her own cultural viewpoint when seeking medical help.

Guidelines for discussing cross-cultural issues

The setting

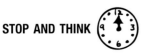

STOP AND THINK

Think back to your first week at medical school. What was it like finding your way around? How did you react to people you didn't know? What was it like having colleagues in the same situation as your own?

The unfamiliar atmosphere and people in a hospital and in other medical settings can make a patient more anxious. It is important that this is respected and that patients are not addressed in a public place. Patients will have their own expectations about their treatment, depending on the setting, e.g. an inpatient hospital raises expectations different from those associated with a GP's surgery. Information about procedures should be made explicit and explained to the patient in order to alleviate any anxiety.

Introductions

There is evidence that doctors communicate differently with patients from ethnic minorities. Because they may not speak English fluently, ethnic-minority patients may also be perceived as less intelligent than the majority culture (and they may also perceive themselves to be less intelligent or competent). Another common occurrence is that the doctor may provide more directive information than would be given to a patient who is fluent and can, therefore, articulate fears and questions easily.

It is important to address patients by the name they prefer and not refer to them in the third person (e.g. 'the Asian gentleman'), thereby depersonalising them. In some cultures, the use of the first name is considered insulting. The doctor can ask questions such as:

"So you are Mr . . . ? Did I pronounce that properly?"

"How do you prefer to be addressed?"

Check that the patient's name is correctly spelled on the records and establish the correct pronunciation. Foreign-sounding names are sometimes seen to be too difficult even to attempt to pronounce: to make no attempt communicates a lack of interest in anything that is different. In geographic areas with a large number of ethnic-minority patients, hospital wards should have a copy of the naming systems used in different cultures. For example, the Muslim and Hindu naming systems are different from that used in western Europe and can cause confusion for patients and their records. In Muslim cultures there are several inherited names. For example, a South-east Asian Muslim man will have a different name from his wife. He may be called Mohammed Ishak – the first name refers to his religious name and the latter to the personal name. They are stated in this order. There is often no family name. Female Muslims have two names also, but the structure is different from males. For example, in the name Fatima Bibi, the first name is the personal one and the second is the equivalent of 'Miss' or 'Madam'. If it is translated, Mrs Bibi means literally 'Mrs Wife'. But you may also find that a Muslim gives his last name as the surname even though this is the personal name, in order to make communication with non-Muslims easier.

Communication may need to be more indirect, avoiding the direct question-and-answer method characteristic of Europe and the USA or at least paced so that one gets a sense of the communication style required.[3] Although patients from these societies may find this style familiar and business-like, patients from other countries may expect to be asked details about their family and may find it strange that the doctor wants to begin the medical interview immediately. For these reasons, it is important to explain explicitly how you will be assessing them:

"I need to ask you some questions about your health. I'll go through them, and I would like you to say 'yes' or 'no' to the questions. Afterwards, we can discuss how you are doing with the treatment and if you have any worries or questions."

Obtaining relevant psychological information

Basic biographical information usually gives clues to further questions that should be asked about the patient's cultural background, e.g. whether the patient was born or brought up in the majority culture, or has just arrived; whether the patient's stay is temporary, or whether the individual intends to reside in this country permanently. Rather than assume that the patient is an immigrant, a temporary resident or of a particular nationality, the doctor should ask instead: 'Would you please tell me where you were born?'

The doctor can avoid imposing meaning on the patient's culture by being open and exploratory in cultural aspects that may be unfamiliar. For example, in a routine check-up, a pregnant Greek-Cypriot woman says she has been fasting. The doctor tries to understand her reasons for not eating a balanced diet before he gives her medical advice:

PATIENT: *I have been fasting for the last 10 days and I feel quite weak.*
DOCTOR: *I'm not sure why you've been fasting?*
PATIENT: *Because it is the Greek Easter this weekend.*
DOCTOR: *Could you tell me more about that? I didn't know that the Greek Easter is at a different time from our own Easter!*

The doctor should focus on finding out about cultural factors relevant to the presenting problem. In the above case, the doctor should ask for how long she plans to continue fasting and may then suggest acceptable foods she could include in her diet without breaking her fast.

Once a patient has disclosed information about cultural preferences, the doctor should acknowledge the significance of these factors to the patient, especially if the patient will be hospitalised (Table 7.1). The doctor could pose general questions such as:

"Is there anything else you'd like to ask about your treatment, or what will happen during your visits (or stay in hospital)?"

"I'm sometimes unsure whether there are specific cultural differences that I should be asking about, so you have to help me along and let me know if there is anything that could be helpful for you."

There may be situations where a particular cultural practice is too elaborate to perform in a busy hospital, so it may be necessary to tell the patient that further negotiation needs to take place first (e.g. with the nurses or ward sister). If cultural practices cannot be accommodated in the hospital, then it is important to explain this to the patient to prevent misunderstanding.

Explore the patient's ideas about the illness

As stated earlier, patients may have their own ideas about the cause of their illness. The doctor can try to understand these ideas by asking questions (Table 7.3). The answers can provide insight into the patient's problem and might help to make appropriate suggestions for the treatment.[4]

Explore the patient's expectations of treatment

The doctor can ask questions such as:

"What kind of treatment do you think you should receive?"

"What are you hoping for from the treatment?"

Table 7.3 Guidelines for exploring the patient's perception of illness, care and treatment

Guidelines	Questions
Explore individual views of the illness, care and treatment	Can you describe to me how you have been feeling? What type of treatment do you think would help? How do you think we should proceed with the treatment?
Does the patient attribute the problem to internal (biological and physiological) factors, or to external (e.g. supernatural, religious) causes?	What do you think is the cause of your illness?
Is the illness expressed psychologically or physiologically?	Could you show me where you feel the illness? What symptoms have you had? When and how did you realise you were unwell?
Does the patient believe he or she has any control over the illness, care and treatment?	What have you done since you found out you were ill?
Are there relatives or friends who have an impact on the patient's life? What is their perception of the illness?	Who advised you to begin this treatment? [*addressing a relative*]: What do you think is the reason your relative has not been well?
Generally, what are the cultural ideas about the illness?	How does your culture view people who have cancer/AIDS?
Is there common ground between the doctor's and the patient's model?	I suggest you take the medication for another few days even though you are feeling better. Do you agree with me?

Illness and its treatment should be explained in terms that will both fit in with the patient's beliefs and acknowledge the doctor's expertise. If cultural differences are irreconcilable, the doctor should acknowledge them, thus demonstrating that the patient's views are not being devalued. After all, patients are free to choose what sort of treatment to accept. For example, during Ramadan, a Muslim patient asked if treatment could be postponed until the religious festival had ended. This was not possible because it was crucial that the treatment should start immediately. In such a case, the doctor needs to explain why treatment must begin at once and help the individual understand that starting the treatment now is for the patient's benefit and not because of a disregard for religious practices. Most religions permit some flexibility in regard to medical treatment when there is a measure of urgency, or in life-and-death situations.

Find a compromise between medical treatment and cultural values

The doctor and patient might have different worldviews, or attitudes, about the following topics:

- spiritual beliefs and practices
- sociocultural ideas
- familial experiences and values
- beliefs about health, illness and treatment
- beliefs and stereotypes about the minority culture.

Some aspects of a patient's lifestyle may sound exotic or bizarre to the doctor, but you should remember that they are part of the patient's cultural values. For example, it may be difficult to understand why a patient wants relatives to be present at all consultations, as in western cultures there is generally more emphasis on individuality and privacy. Similarly, the doctor's values may seem abnormal to the patient. In cross-cultural communication, the doctor must begin by establishing a rapport before proceeding with the treatment. Your aim should be to decrease the cultural distance between your worldview as the doctor and the patient's worldview. You should not impose your own cultural attitudes on the patient but, rather, work to create common ground in relation to the treatment (Fig. 7.1).This common ground can be negotiated taking into consideration the patient's needs and cultural background and the hospital context and treatment requirements.

Consult relatives

There may be times when it is helpful to consult the relatives of a patient to obtain more information about the family's practices in the management of the patient's illness. In dealing with emotive areas such as death in the family, the relatives need to be consulted on

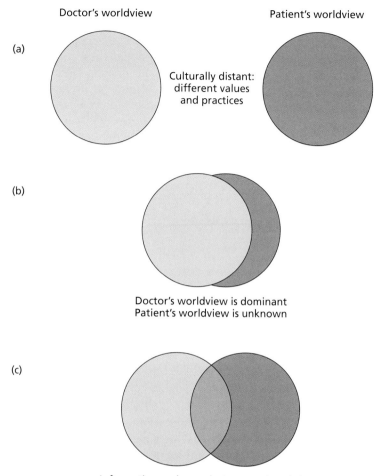

Fig. 7.1 Working to create common ground in relation to treatment.

culturally appropriate practices. For example, in Judaism, the deceased must be buried as soon as possible, usually within 24 hours, and mutilation of the body is not allowed unless there is a legal requirement for a post-mortem. For Hindus, the dying patient is usually read passages from the Holy Book, and once the person has died the body must be left uncovered. The rituals surrounding death are emotive ones for the relatives, and to make decisions without consulting them could be viewed as offensive and disrespectful.

The use of interpreters

The use of interpreters is commonplace in most health care settings. If the patient or relatives speak little or no English, it is best to consult interpreters to make sure the relatives understand the nature of the illness and the treatment planned. They also need to be given an opportunity to ask questions. Translators are also important even for patients with a little knowledge of English, for it can be a relief for patients to speak their native language. Moreover, an interpreter from the patient's own culture can identify crucial issues and give comfort and support. When an interpreter is present, the doctor should aim to develop a rapport with both the interpreter and the patient. However, there can be problems in using interpreters in medical consultations.

Some problems in using interpreters

- There is the possibility of bias when communication is dependent on a third party.
- Meanings can be changed in the process of translation.
- Interpreters are often lay people and are not usually familiar with medical terminology, so clear communication is inhibited.
- An interpreter's presence may embarrass the patient when the problem is perceived as a taboo subject (e.g. a sexual problem), especially if the interpreter is of the same nationality.
- An interpreter might reinterpret the patient's ideas or abbreviate responses, as sometimes the interpreter will have his or her own ideas and biases about treatment. This can annoy doctors who are trying to open up communication and learn more. The translator can be a help but also a hindrance! Ideally, well-trained interpreters, or those who are used to the health care setting, should be consulted.

Consult colleagues

Sometimes it may be necessary to consult colleagues in order to find the most effective way of bridging cross-cultural differences and the hospital practices. Colleagues of the same cultural background as the patient may be particularly helpful in suggesting ways to ensure that the patient feels supported (e.g. they can provide the presence of someone who speaks the patient's language).

The use of other social networks

The patient should be made aware of the variety of useful resources available to people from different cultures, such as counselling services, ethnic centres and other culturally specific information. Networks or community support may be the most helpful for patients and their family. For many countries the biomedical model is not the most prominent healing system, so other types of support could be consulted, such as traditional faith healers and herbalists. Members of some religious groups may want to consult a minister of religion to perform religious rites. Details of such groups should be kept on each ward and given to patients who request them. It is important to leave time for the patient to discuss other questions or concerns.

Case example 7.2

A female Arab patient on the ward

Mahmooda, aged 43 years, with three children, was suffering from cancer and was hospitalised for several months when her condition deteriorated. She found being in hospital particularly difficult, and her only comfort was prayer. However, because she usually got up to pray at night, she woke up the other patients, who then complained to the nurses. When a nurse tried to talk to her the next day, she would not listen and continued to get up at night to pray. The nurse spoke to the doctor, who suggested that an interpreter working in the hospital could come along to talk to the patient and the doctor. Through the interpreter, the doctor explained the problem without being judgemental:

DOCTOR: *I understand that you've been getting up to pray at night and that the other patients have complained about being woken up. I wonder if we can find a way for you to be able to do this at a time when you will not wake up the others?*

MAHMOODA: *Tell the doctor that I need to pray. I am ill – look at how I have changed. I am like an old woman now.*

DOCTOR: *I know it's been very difficult for you in the last few weeks; you've had a lot to cope with.*

The patient was silent for a few minutes. The doctor also remained silent and then asked her how she had been getting on with the medication.

MAHMOODA: *I've found it all very difficult and I miss my children. You know, I can't take care of them now. It really breaks my heart.*

The doctor nodded and then asked whether her children had been able to come and visit her. Mahmooda's face lit up:

MAHMOODA: *Yes, my little one came yesterday with my two older ones. Usually, it's the older ones who come so that their father stays to look after the younger one. You know, she's too young, and it upsets her to see me here. It upsets all of us, it upsets me that they have to see their mother this way [cries].*

The doctor then asked her about her praying and acknowledged the importance of the act of prayer for her.

DOCTOR: *It seems to be your source of comfort to pray when you are on your own at night.*

MAHMOODA: *Yes, it is. I don't know what I would do if I didn't have faith.*

DOCTOR: *Mahmooda, I know it's important for you to be able to pray, and that is why we need to find a way for you to say your prayers and yet be sure the other patients are not awakened.*

MAHMOODA: *I don't see how. It's the only time I am alone and I can concentrate.*

DOCTOR: *Well, perhaps you can be alone at other times and pray then. There is a relatives' room nearby which often remains empty. Do you think you could go and have a look, and if you find it suitable, perhaps you can do your prayers there? This way, you can have your privacy and the other patients are not disturbed at night.*

MAHMOODA: *But I don't know where it is.*

The interpreter explained that she would show her where the room was and that they would find out when it was not in use by others so that Mahmooda could have privacy for her prayers.

Different services, treatments and doctors will hold a different status across cultures. When working with people from different cultures, credibility issues need to be addressed whenever possible. In some cultures the doctor holds a lower status if female.

In the case example above, the doctor shows sensitivity towards the patient's different cultural practices (Table 7.2). Sensitivity also needs to be shown when medically examining a Muslim woman. Especially with a gynaecological examination, it is usual for Muslim women to request a female doctor. In the case of Mahmooda, although the doctor is male, he manages to show her respect by acknowledging her distress at being in hospital. At the same time, he is politely explicit about what she can and cannot do in hospital.

Case example 7.3

Asian female seeking urgent medical consultation

Shereen, a 17-year-old Indian girl, has been admitted to casualty with abdominal pains. She has pain but does not want to be examined by a male doctor, and her father insists that they would like to see a female doctor. The nurse acknowledges their wish, but explains that this is impossible, as the only doctor covering the casualty department is male.

If the family feel respected and are given the opportunity, they can provide reasons for their cultural demands. These can help the staff find out if anything can be done to meet the family's needs. In this case, the family also feel exposed and do not wish to discuss the problem in the casualty waiting area. Realising this, the nurse finds a quiet place where they can talk in private.

FATHER: *It is not religiously correct for a man to touch our daughter, do you understand? It is only her husband who is allowed to touch her after they are married.*

NURSE: *I'm afraid the only doctor on duty is male. May I explain to you that it is normal practice in our hospital that when a woman has to be examined for gynaecological concerns, then a female nurse has to be present in the room. Do you think this would be acceptable to you and make it easier for your daughter?*

The nurse makes this suggestion tentatively so that the family does not feel that a solution is imposed on them. They can refuse medical treatment if they feel they have to compromise their cultural or religious beliefs too much. In this case, the girl is in considerable pain, and cultural values have to be compromised. She agrees to be examined by the male doctor, but asks not to have to undress in front of him and for the nurse to be present as well. She allows her father to do all the communicating with the doctor.

In the side room, the girl is left alone with the nurse. The nurse asks Shereen how she is feeling and tries to develop a relationship with her – this can prove crucial to the examination and to the girl's willingness to comply with treatment:

> NURSE: *What do you think is wrong? Can you tell me where it hurts so I can tell the doctor?*
> SHEREEN: *Well, I seem to have a pain here [points to her abdomen]. See?*
> NURSE: *Can you show me exactly where it hurts?*

The girl shows the nurse more clearly and asks whether she has to show the doctor, as well. The nurse replies that it would be helpful because they need to have his opinion so they can do something to get rid of her pain. The girl changes into a hospital robe, but is allowed to keep her shirt underneath to cover her back and arms. Meanwhile the nurse continues to build up her relationship with the girl, enquiring about her siblings. When they enter the room the doctor introduces himself. He is aware of the issues and acknowledges them.

> DOCTOR: *I'm sorry that your daughter has to be examined by a man, but I'm afraid I am the only doctor on duty tonight. I think she needs to be seen straight away since she is in pain, so I shall have to examine her myself. I really think we have no choice at this stage. If possible, we can try to arrange for a female doctor to follow up, if that is necessary.*

The family is given the choice, but at the same time the doctor lets them know that he takes the cultural issues and their daughter's health seriously. The doctor then asks questions and the father replies on behalf of his daughter:

> DOCTOR: *When did the pains start?*
> FATHER: *They started this morning and then they got worse.*

The doctor confirms this with the girl by communicating with the nurse. It is important to do this, because under stress, relatives can convey the wrong information in their attempt to be helpful. It is appropriate that the doctor then focuses on the parents' concerns about the possible diagnosis, emphasising that this is only an investigative stage and that he cannot be sure.

The family is anxious to know if there are gynaecological problems and need clarification about the diagnosis. They are concerned about their daughter's ability to bear children and need further reassurance. The doctor knows that it is important to address their concerns while being honest about the possible treatment, in case the girl is found to have a cyst. The doctor needs to clarify the following areas:

● Who will be attending the next appointment with the girl?
● How do they feel about seeing him again? Would they prefer him to arrange a referral to a female colleague?
● How much has the family understood about the medical procedures? (He does not want them to leave the hospital with unnecessary anxiety.)
● Will it be necessary to bring a translator to explain the medical details thoroughly?
● What are the family's feelings about a translator from the same community? (Gynaecology and child-bearing are sensitive subjects.)
● Should he now give the family more information about the possible consequences if a cyst is found, or wait until further meetings?

> DOCTOR: *I feel it may be appropriate for Shereen to speak to the nurse now about how to manage in the next few weeks if she experiences further pain, and about how to identify other symptoms. If you prefer, the next time you come we can arrange for you to have an appointment with a female doctor.*

The doctor tells the family what they can expect, while in another room Shereen and the nurse review the details to make sure that Shereen has understood and has a chance to ask questions. The nurse confirms her next appointment.

> SHEREEN: *Will you be here next time I come to hospital?*
> NURSE: *I'm on duty that day, but in case I become involved in something I can't leave, we will make sure that another female nurse can be with you when you see the doctor. I will also try to be free for your appointment in 3 weeks' time.*

Case example 7.4

Refugee family from Afghanistan seeking advice regarding their son's health

This family has been in the UK for a period of less than a year. During this time they had a baby boy, Hussein. They have two older girls and have longed for a boy. Since he was born shortly after fleeing Afghanistan they have always been concerned about his health. Their health visitor has voiced some concerns regarding the baby's development. Since she is one of the few people they have regular contact with they become confused and distressed about her comments, but the father does not feel in a position to discuss these matters with her. This is a common example as it demonstrates how often doctors' consulting rooms can become the only arena for cross-cultural conflicts regarding health to be addressed.

DOCTOR: *Tell me about your concerns for the baby [at this stage nearly 1 year].*

FATHER: *I am sure he is fine. We just came to you for advice.*

DOCTOR: *What advice can I help with?*

FATHER: *The nurse was worried about the baby's not growing normally.*

DOCTOR: *I am wondering if you have the same concerns as your health visitor does for the baby.*

FATHER: *Maybe our baby is different in some way ... [hesitates and then when asked to be specific, turns to the mother for more information. Although she understands most of the exchange, she responds in their language and the father translates for the doctor].*

FATHER: *The nurse felt that he was not moving enough and about his diet.*

In this case much of the conflict was due to cultural factors and different expectations on development. As this was a third child who was a baby boy the father was particularly anxious that the implication of the health visitor was that his son had some type of brain damage. The doctor decided it would be useful to assess the baby, but to do so at a time when a translator would be present. Even though the father's English was good enough, there were many words inappropriately used. Also, the patient did not seem to understand fully the term 'health visitor' or what her role involved. The health visitor's main concern was that the baby was not as mobile as he ought to be for his age, and that he was not exploring enough or being 'allowed to become independent'. Furthermore, she was concerned that the mother breast-fed him but provided no other supplements.

From the onset, in many cultures it is the mother who determines the infant's physical space and exploration space. This aspect is largely culturally defined,[5] even as far as what is considered a safe distance to move away from others. The mother did not attend any playgroups and was rather cautious after their experiences in Afghanistan, fearing that something might happen to the baby (this emerged much later in the discussion).

In this case there are many learning points, taking into account the whole family's perspective. For example, in this case, it is the mother who knows the child best and speaking to her through an interpreter was helpful. The father takes the role of narrator and also translator, which implies at times that it is difficult for the doctor to assess carefully the baby's development and understand his use of language. Additionally, when there are cross-cultural conflicts, it is useful for the doctor to communicate to the health visitor or other professionals involved as to how cultural factors (or the impact of trauma in the case of refugees, especially political refugees) may play a role. In the case of Hussein's family, being new arrivals to the country, they were anxious for the health of their son. The doctor (female in this case) is held in esteem by this family, as in their country women would be much less likely to become doctors. The examination and assessment of the baby were carried out and he was found to be normal. The family were able to discuss alternatives to the child's diet and physical needs, finding a way to provide what was necessary for his continued normal development and, at the same time, respecting their cultural preferences and beliefs. The mother was happy to continue breast-feeding once a day and providing the baby with additional solid food during the day.

Another consideration when working with refugee patients is that laws are in constant flux as to what treatment they are entitled to receive and at which point of their immigration process. This again provides a sensitive issue for families at a time of physical ill health and uncertainty for medical staff regarding the extent and follow-up possibilities in terms of treatment. Clarification of these issues may mean more realistic treatment options or alter the treatment plan in some cases.

Key points

- It is important to allow patients to explain their cultural background, values, beliefs and expectations when these may be relevant to the consultation.
- Heightened awareness of cultural issues can help you to make a more accurate assessment of the patient's behaviour, to improve the therapeutic relationship and to enhance treatment.
- There are certain cultural groups, particularly new arrivals or refugees, that may have multiple psychological and physical concerns and these may need to be discussed when there is a sense of trust and safety, i.e. assessment may take longer than with someone with full command of the language, culture and system.
- The doctor needs to accept other people's cultural and racial ideas as different, but equally important.
- Important issues can be overlooked if either the doctor or the patient fears misunderstanding and rejection of cultural values.
- The patient may be part of a particular culture, but will have adopted some aspects of it and rejected others. The doctor must carefully assess each patient's individual and cultural needs before deciding on an appropriate treatment.
- Matching patient and doctor according to race or culture is not always helpful or necessarily desirable.

FURTHER READING

Berry WJ, Poortinga YH, Segall MH et al 2002 Cross-cultural psychology: research and applications. Cambridge University Press, Cambridge

Eleftheriadou Z 1994 Transcultural counselling. Central Books, London

Kleinman A 1980 Patients and healers in the context of culture. University of California Press, Berkeley

REFERENCES

1. Helman CG 2000 Culture, health and illness. Hodder Arnold, London
2. Mullavey-O'Byrne C 1994 Intercultural communication for health care doctors. In: Brislin RW, Yoshida T (eds) 1994 Improving intercultural interactions: modules for cross-cultural training programmes. Sage, London
3. Neuliep JW 2006 Intercultural communication: a contextual approach, 3rd edn. Sage, London
4. Gardiner HW, Kosmitzki C 2004 Lives across cultures. Allyn & Bacon, Columbus, OH, USA
5. Brislin RW, Yoshida T (eds) 1994 Improving intercultural interactions: modules for cross-cultural training programmes. Sage, London

8

Guidelines on communicating with children and young people

Co-written by Zack Eleftheriadou

Management of children

Although children may suffer similar medical problems to those of adults, their management in the clinical setting is, of necessity, different in certain respects. Some doctors welcome the challenge of caring for sick children whereas others are reluctant and, where possible, avoid the situation. Working with children offers rewards as well as many challenges (Table 8.1).

Table 8.1 What makes caring for children difficult?

- Not knowing what to say to a child, or how to say it without using complex medical language
- The child's fear or anxiety in the presence of a stranger: the child may be silent, or cry
- A child's previous unpleasant experience of illness may make him or her unmanageable or difficult to examine
- In pain, children may scream and wriggle
- You may fear hurting the child
- Difficulty with procedures (e.g. taking blood) can make the doctor frustrated and irritable
- The parents may be difficult to deal with
- The child might need to be separated from his or her parents
- Parents may be overwhelmed by a fear of losing their child
- If there are signs of abuse or deprivation, the doctor may feel uncertain about broaching the subject

---

Modes of communication (Table 8.2)

Verbal interaction

Care must be taken when communicating with children to ensure that the conversation is pitched at the child's cognitive level, and that the

---

Table 8.2 Improving your communication with child patients

Do

- Put yourself at the same physical level as the child when you examine or talk to him or her
- Establish rapport before touching or examining a child; gain the child's confidence
- Learn the child's terminology for his or her concerns and parts of the anatomy
- Explain procedures before you do them. Prepare the child for a strange noise or smell, a painful procedure or change from a familiar routine
- Keep talking. A calm voice is reassuring, even if it doesn't stop the child crying
- Engage the help of a parent or guardian, especially when examining a child

Don't

- Rely too much on bribery or small gifts. The child will constantly expect a reward after treatment or medication. You can also create a state of dependence that will be hard to reverse
- Make promises you can't keep, e.g. 'this won't hurt'. False reassurance can make a child confused, depressed or unmanageable
- Use complex language or medical terms. If appropriate, check the child's understanding by asking the child to repeat what you have said, or to demonstrate using a doll or teddy bear
- Allow the child to worry about a medical procedure. Try to carry it out immediately to prevent prolonged anxiety
- Leave the child alone in an unfamiliar setting or with unfamiliar people
- Encourage the child to be 'good'. Instead, give the child permission to cry or scream

---

pace corresponds to developmental changes. Children and young people also undergo changes that may influence their emotional response during and after treatment. It is important to check whether the child has understood what has been said. Children pick up subtle cues from both the doctor and their parents, so there should be as much consistency as possible. It has been shown that young patients are less anxious if told what is likely to happen to them and if this is explained clearly and honestly. Explanations like this will also improve rapport between the doctor and the child. Children find it useful to know the exact sequence of events and may ask repeatedly about the order of events. There may be a need for follow-up consults with children and young people (particularly when parents are not supporting or do not understand the treatment details) so that the correct technique is maintained (for example, in terms of asthma management).

Role of play and drawings

Young children sometimes find it easier to express their concerns about illness and treatment through play rather than through conversation alone. Where practicable, parents should be asked to bring to the consultation a favourite toy or other object that will facilitate communicating with the child. If the toys used are the child's own, the child will identify with them more readily. If however, the child has not brought in any toys, some should be available in a play area. It is important to ensure that care is child-centred. Toys help to establish rapport with children. They can also be used to explain medical procedures and to gather important clues about the child's mastery of cognitive tasks. Animal toys, puppets, teddy bears and dolls can be very useful, for example:

> *"Shall we have a look at teddy's tummy and find out where it hurts? What would teddy need to make him feel better?"*

> *"Show panda how wide you can open your mouth."*

The physical environment

STOP AND THINK 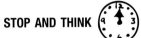 *Adults take for granted that our physical environment is built in proportion with ourselves and not children. Look around you wherever you happen to be now: if you were half or a third your size, what would become an obstacle?*

- *Could you still reach the door handle?*
- *Could you climb up on a chair, or would you need to be lifted up?*
- *Could you sit at a table and still put your elbows on it?*
- *Could you get up or down stairs on your own?*
- *Could you leave where you are now without help from an adult?*

Obviously it is not possible to create a totally child-oriented environment in all settings, but think about the future when you are qualified. If you are a GP or work in a hospital, what would you want to do to make sure young patients felt more welcome and comfortable where you work?

Play materials and the play area

Access to a well-equipped play area and toys in the waiting room show that the environment is child-oriented. Children find it comforting to see brightly coloured walls, play materials and furniture (e.g. small tables and chairs) that are in scale with their size. Some children's hospitals name wards after animals and ensure that door handles and other objects are at a level that can be easily reached by most children. On the other hand, consideration must be given to safety. Toys should be selected accordingly and children should not be allowed to leave the area or ward unescorted. Most hospitals now also have a playroom that is to be used for inpatient mobile children staffed with a playleader. Playleaders have experience working with children in hospital and will select appropriate toys for them. This is a very important attempt to normalise the setting as much as possible and create fun distractions. Toys and the familiarity of a children's room give the child a sense of control. For those children who are confined to their bed the playleader will make visits to the children and bring them toys. The toys give a bridging language for the child and health professional.

Doctors' appearance

The dress and appearance of doctors can help a child to feel comfortable in hospital. Some doctors have multicoloured stethoscopes, wear fun badges on their lapels and carry a small, fluffy toy in their pocket in case a child needs to be distracted or cheered up. Many dispense with uniforms or white coats, or wear casual clothes, in order to create a more relaxed and friendly impression. Wherever possible, the preferences of the child/adolescent and/or his or her parent or guardian should be taken into consideration. This may also mean that care should be coordinated across the whole of the hospital/health organisation and be available as close to the patient's home as possible (for example, this applies especially to children and young people with cancer). All the above factors may improve the rapport with the doctor and increase the likelihood of good compliance with hospital attendance and medical procedures.

The consulting room

Like the waiting room, the consulting room ought to be child-oriented. Remember that children need privacy just as much as adults, so if they need to be examined, be sure to draw the curtains or shut the door. Often extra consultation time needs to be booked in when working with children and young people.

Introductions

You should be flexible in your ability to interact appropriately with children at their different stages of development. You also need to be able to differentiate between normal development and a developmental delay that may require special attention. Each stage in child development has its own milestones and conflicts. Some children build up trust slowly, so if a child is initially shy, it is important to persevere. Ask about hobbies and interests before addressing medical problems.

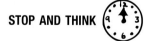 **STOP AND THINK** *There are many textbooks on child development, but common sense and intuition work best in communicating successfully with children. Think how you would explain human reproduction to a 3-year-old, a 4-year-old, an 8-year-old and a 12-year-old.*

Try this with a friend or another student. Listen to the words each of you chooses. Do you sound childish? Overly scientific and complex? Patronising? Do you lecture, draw, use puppets or dolls? Do you ask the 'child' questions to check the child's level of understanding and knowledge of familiar terms for parts of the body?

Gathering information about the patient

Conversation with an infant is impossible, even though the doctor can talk to both the infant and parents. This presents a challenge in history-taking. Infants have their own personality and preferences and the most effective way of learning about these is to interact, e.g. make eye contact; lean towards the baby at a safe enough distance not to seem threatening, but close enough for the baby to see you clearly; speak to the baby in a calm, gentle manner. If the infant looks playful, you may find yourself smiling more and making quick, high-toned sounds; if the infant looks serious, you should change your manner accordingly.

In this way you can gather information about the baby's temperament, how it is pacified and how it soothes itself (e.g. thumb-sucking) and how it interacts (e.g. smiling or vocalising patterns). As the check-up proceeds, you should give the parents feedback on the baby's stage of development. This is the time when parents are likely to voice their own concerns about their baby or about their general abilities as parents. For example:

> Dr Richard: *She's got a strong grip. And look, she's already trying to turn herself over. Soon she will be crawling.*
>
> Mrs Katz: *But why doesn't she like to be held by her father?*
>
> Dr Richard: *Babies often get more used to one parent. It may need some time. She seems to prefer to be held like this. Perhaps you can encourage her dad to do that.*

Parents continually compare their child's development with other children and their own norms, and often seek reassurance, particularly from a doctor. It is a good idea to explain that there is no right or wrong way to bring up a child, and that it is not always useful to make comparisons about development.

Addressing the child

It is important not to talk down to children. If communication is pitched at an age level younger than the child, that child will feel you are not taking him or her seriously. Being addressed appropriately (similarly to any informational leaflets which can be written specifically for children) makes children feel reassured that they will be understood and respected. This can determine how comfortable they feel about sharing questions and fears. The doctor can try to create a rapport by asking about favourite hobbies, school and friends. If the child shows independence from his or her parents, ask if the child want to be examined whilst sitting on mother's lap or on the examining table. Some children build up trust slowly, so if a child seems shy it is important not to appear threatening. This is more applicable to young children who may not want to be moved from a parent's lap. The doctor might say: 'You don't want to move away from mummy? That's fine. You can stand right next to her if you like'.

Judge how comfortable the child feels by the way the child walks into the consulting room. For example, does the child stride in front of the parents, or refuse to leave mother's side? This might be the child's characteristic way of meeting new people, or the child may be anxious about the unfamiliar setting. You should take some time to establish rapport before starting the examination or asking medical questions.[1] Make the encounter feel like a collaborative activity by inviting the child and parents to participate in decision-making. Children are more likely to take an interest in their treatment, and to trust the doctor and want to return, if they feel involved and have some control in the medical encounter. The doctor might say: 'Let's see, what do you think we should do to get rid of this?'

It is helpful to engage the support of the parent when talking to and examining a child. Some parents feel extremely guilty about having to seek the help of professionals when there is a concern about their child's health. The doctor can try to reassure them and increase their confidence by praising the positive aspects of their relationship. It is essential that the child be viewed as an individual with needs distinct from those of the parents.

Addressing the child's feelings

The hospital environment can cause anxiety in children, and their behaviour may regress to that of a much younger child. This is quite normal, but by addressing the child's feelings, e.g. of fear, loss, abandonment or disability, you can help maintain self-esteem and prevent some behavioural problems. You may have to respond to something that you sense the child is communicating but has not verbalised clearly.

After each medical procedure, you should compliment, congratulate or encourage children before preparing them for the next stage. Children may blame themselves for an illness, believing that it is a punishment for bad behaviour. Children can believe this so strongly that they become negative and stubborn in order to prove that they have done something wrong and that they deserve to be punished. You should reassure children that sickness is not the result of naughtiness and that they are not responsible for the illness, e.g.:

> "This is something that happens to other children too, not just to you, so you mustn't feel it's your fault. I've seen lots of other children with broken arms. Let me explain what we have to do."

A child needs to have the opportunity to explore feelings and ask questions about medical procedures. Children who fully recover can be made to feel they have mastered the illness, and chronically ill children need to be repeatedly told how well they are coping and that they can still fight the illness. Children also like to feel in control and that they have acquired new skills regarding their illness. For example, a child might learn to detect some warning signals and in turn inform the parents. Even when the procedures are over, the child can be encouraged to articulate or play out medical procedures that have made a particular impression. On some wards it has been useful to have photo albums of procedures that the children view together with the relevant professional before a procedure. This provides information for the children, shows them that other children have been through a similar experience and gives them, and the parents, the opportunity to visualise what might happen, or even to return to it at a later stage.

Dealing with adolescents

Adolescence is a time of physiological, cognitive and psychological changes. Adolescents need time to understand and integrate all the enormous changes taking place in the period between childhood and adulthood. In some areas they may be able to make decisions like an adult, and in others they may feel unsure and child-like. Trying to adjust to the changes (such as changing appearance, different bodily sensations and odour, intense emotions and fluctuating moods, and different responsibilities/roles as well as reactions from people) can be difficult, and coping with medical concerns can cause more problems. Special care has to be taken to be respectful to this changing body and role. As the doctor, you have to show that you are on their side and are prepared to be open in response to their concerns and anxieties. Adolescents need boundaries – perhaps even more than children do – but they will often test these to the limit. For example, they may arrive late at the consultation or not attend at all, or not comply with the treatment.

The doctor needs to find creative ways to give adolescents choices. Even if there are minor choices to make in terms of the actual medical treatment, there may be small areas that can be negotiated; for example, who comes with them or where they sit for their consult. It really does matter and will make them feel they have some control. This is particularly significant as they are already coping with bodily changes and their body might feel 'foreign'. If the body is also probed medically or with unnecessary or thoughtless questioning then this feeling can intensify.

The doctor's task is a delicate one because the boundaries need to be flexible. You have to take into account different individuals and circumstances, but at the same time you must be prepared to confront the adolescent when appropriate, e.g. acknowledge the adolescent's desire to be independent, but emphasise the importance of attending appointments. Other adolescents may have a sense of omnipotence and sometimes take risks, such as having unprotected sexual intercourse. Your role is to explain the dangers and possible consequences of their actions, particularly when parents or teachers have failed to do so. You should also provide an opportunity for them to air their concerns, while taking care not to lecture them. Some of these points are illustrated in the case of George (Case example 8.1).

Case example 8.1

Anaemic adolescent refusing treatment

George, a Greek-Cypriot boy in his early teens, has thalassaemia major, a type of anaemia found in Mediterranean populations. He needs blood transfusions every 4 weeks, as a result of which his body builds up excess iron. To get rid of the iron, he needs continuous infusion of a chelating agent via a pump 5 days a week. He does not mind the transfusions or hospital visits because he meets other young people with thalassaemia, but in the last few weeks he has begun to resent having to use the pump, and during his routine check his iron level was found to be high. Worried about the result, his parents brought him to the hospital. The doctor feels that because the boy is so silent, the doctor and George should talk in private so George can have the opportunity to ask questions he might not wish to ask in front of his anxious parents.

DR NORTON: *I understand you've found it difficult to use the pump recently, and the tests show that your iron level has increased.*

GEORGE: *Yeah – I know.*

The doctor needs to make sure that George understands what the results mean:

DR NORTON: *Am I right in assuming you have seen your test results? [George nods.] I'll go through the results with you and then perhaps we can talk about the treatment.*

GEORGE: *I know about the treatment, but I'm just so sick of it.*

DR NORTON: *I know you are, and I know your parents have been really concerned.*

GEORGE: *Yeah, they came with me today to make you convince me to take my treatment.*

DR NORTON: *You know that at the end of the day it's your decision what you do, but I'd like us to talk about the treatment and see what we can negotiate. You're obviously aware that the iron levels in your blood are too high at the moment, and we need to get rid of it now when you're still in the early stages of your development.*

GEORGE: *What do you mean? That I still have time to live?*

DR NORTON: *What I mean is that because your body is going through a great deal of development during adolescence, if the iron removal is consistent, you have a much better chance of developing normally. If the excess iron is not removed, it can accumulate in the blood and stunt your development. This can result in you looking much younger than your age.*

GEORGE: *Yeah, I've seen people like that at the hospital – it's really frightening!*

DR NORTON: *I need to explain that you won't die if you don't take the treatment in the short term. But if the build-up of iron is prolonged, then body organs can be damaged and this can lead to complications. So the iron overload takes some time to accumulate – it doesn't build up in a few days – and that's why the earlier we treat it, the better the outcome for you.*

GEORGE: *So it doesn't matter that I haven't used the pump the last few weeks?*

DR NORTON: *Well, you're not in a serious situation, but at the same time we need to monitor the iron level to prevent further accumulation. The treatment should help the level drop to normal again. George, I know it's frustrating for you to have to use the pump so many days of the week, and it does get awkward when you have to explain it to your friends, especially when you want to go out, but it's a small price to pay when you can prevent other complications arising.*

GEORGE: *So if I take the treatment I'll develop normally?*

DR NORTON: *If you take the treatment consistently, you've got a much better chance of developing normally. How do you feel about trying to go back to the treatment?*

GEORGE: *I'm not sure. I just hate getting nagged by my parents – as if I were a child. Anyway, it's really embarrassing to have the pump when I'm with friends.*

DR NORTON: *You can show your parents that they don't need to treat you like a child if you take responsibility for your own body. After all, it does belong to you. As for your friends, I can understand how it may feel embarrassing, but if they're really good friends, you could explain why you have to have the treatment. Do you think they would understand?*

GEORGE: *I don't know – I never really thought of telling them, but I'll think about it.*

DR NORTON: *We've got a few minutes left. Would you like to ask me any other questions?*

The example shows that when George has time alone with the doctor, he can express his own concerns: his anxiety about his health; his fear of dying; his irritation that because his parents worry so much they do not allow him to take decisions; and his embarrassment about having the treatment when his friends are around. The doctor acknowledges his concerns and treats him like an adult, giving him the facts and the chance to ask questions. Don't assume that adolescents will have their questions ready. It may be beneficial for young people to be encouraged to ask questions and even to arrange a follow-up meeting to encourage reflection and queries to emerge. When working with adolescents, doctors must decide when it is best to see them on their own, with their parents, or with other adolescents who have similar problems.

Separation, isolation and chronic illness

Some medical procedures require a child to be separated from family, friends and familiar environment. A child undergoing a bone marrow transplant, radiotherapy or treatment for an infectious disease may need to spend long periods in hospital. A broken leg may result in confinement and restrictions on movement. Changes to physical appearance will seriously disrupt normal routines and relationships.

These are among the most difficult psychological problems to manage in medicine. The vulnerability of the child, coupled with a loss of the expectations of a normal life, can make working with some children stressful for doctors. Children can be helped if there is consistency in their routine and in the staff who care for them. They often become dependent on their favourite doctor and can become upset if the doctor leaves. Try to inform children of staffing changes, and introduce them to new staff and their roles at the earliest opportunity.

You can help children hospitalised for a long time to adjust to the strange environment by adapting (as much as possible) to their usual routines for meals, baths, etc., and by encouraging them to bring in favourite objects from their room at home. Some hospitals have teachers who visit children and bring schoolwork: it is important for children to gain a sense of achievement and experience progress at a time when their body has let them down. Most important, the child should be helped to feel in control of the environment, whatever limitations are placed on moving outside it. This can be achieved as follows:

- Provide lots of activities, and let the child choose from these.
- Mark and celebrate events, e.g. birthdays, end of term.
- If possible, provide a telephone so that the child can keep in regular contact with friends and family.
- Encourage frequent visits (even if they are short), when possible.
- Encourage the parents and child to put up photographs and pictures so that they feel they have some space that is theirs.
- Encourage the child to make a chart and mark off the days until discharge.
- Where possible, avoid wearing a white coat – dress casually.
- Spend time with the child, even when there are no medical procedures to carry out.
- Give realistic hope.

Breaking bad news to children

Whatever difficulties exist in breaking bad news to adults, they are compounded when dealing with children, even though the task is often more simple and straightforward. For both parents and child, bad news will shatter hopes and dreams about the child's future. A shortened lifespan, chronic illness, disability or death before one's parents are major disruptions that give rise to feelings of shock, disbelief, anger, guilt and blame. Even though the child may adjust relatively quickly to limitations resulting from illness or injury, the parents' distress and the reactions of others may continue to cause upset.

For parents, the painful emotions and reactions arise from:

- fear of loss
- concern about others' reactions
- worry about the child's (and the carer's) quality of life
- loss of developmental milestones.

Both the doctor and the parents eventually have to decide how to tell the child the bad news, and exactly what to say. Even when a child is thought too young to be told, some facts may be impossible to withhold as the child grows older. If children find out unexpectedly about their illness and have not been gradually introduced to it, they can feel angry and cheated. Judge carefully how much information should be given, at which stage and by whom (Table 8.3).

Table 8.3 How to break bad news to children

1. Adapt what you say to the child's age, developmental stage and level of understanding
2. Discuss with parents whether to tell the child, who should tell and what to tell. Respect parents' values; do not go over their heads
3. Try to learn what the child knows about illness and death. Ask about previous experiences in the family or among pets
4. Be direct and honest. Avoid euphemisms. Do not lie. Do not give false reassurance
5. Give explanations in the presence of parents. Repeat information and check what the child has understood
6. Check what meaning the child attaches to explanations so as to avoid misunderstandings and unnecessary anxiety
7. Play, drawings and psychotherapy can help a child to understand disability and loss. Consult experts in these fields
8. Attend to the needs and concerns of parents and siblings, who are sometimes more distressed than the child
9. Accept that a bad temper and tantrums are normal reactions in a severely ill child
10. Emphasise what the child will be able to do, thereby giving realistic hope

The conversation with either the child or parents should cover:

- basic information
- behavioural aspects, or consequences of the information
- the effects this may have on relationships
- the beliefs about the problem.

Such a conversation is illustrated in Figure 8.1, which shows these levels of communication at work in a conversation with a 6-year-old.

Liaising with parents and other professionals

Parents (Table 8.4)

Doctors today have a great deal of responsibility to families and children. You may be a crucial source of advice and support for parents, whereas in the past your role might have been taken by their own parents or other relatives. Sometimes being in the presence of an authority figure can relieve the parents of feelings of responsibility and helplessness in dealing with a sick child. At the same time, current concerns about child sexual abuse may complicate your relationship with the family: the doctor's loyalty must be divided between the child's family, society and the legal system.

Whereas paediatricians often choose their specialty because they enjoy working with children and can easily identify with a child's needs, doctors in other specialties may need to learn how to develop a rapport with parents and maintain the child's confidence. Yet parents also have an important role in preparing the child for clinic or hospital visits. Ideally, both parents should come to the consultation in order to create a family atmosphere. Even if one parent cannot attend, the invitation

(1) Information or statements
Doctor: *'We will need you to come into hospital for a few days so we can find out why your legs feel like jelly.'*

(2) Behaviour in relation to statements
Doctor: *'Have you stayed in hospital before?'*
Child: *'No.'*
Doctor: *'What would you like to bring with you?'*

(3) Effect on relationships
Child: *'I don't want to be without Mummy.'*
Doctor: *'That's all right. Mummy can stay here with you. Who else will you miss?'*
Child: *'Not my brother. He always fights with me. But who will feed my goldfish?'*

(4) Beliefs and fears
Child: *'Will I get better?'*
Doctor: *'I hope so. We all hope you will. But we have to find out what's wrong first.'*
Child: *'My granny died in hospital.'*
Doctor: *'Sometimes people get very sick and they can die. Are you worried you might die?'*
Child: *[looks to mother]*
Mother: *'You'll be fine, my darling.' [tearful]*
Child: *[looks down]*
Doctor: *'Many people worry a lot when they come into hospital. What will help you to worry a little less?'*
Child: *'I want to see where I will be sleeping.'*

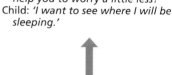

Fig. 8.1 Levels of communication with a child patient.

Table 8.4 Guidelines for helping parents manage their sick child

- Invite both parents to see the doctor to get factual information
- Make them feel involved; acknowledge their expertise as parents
- Be honest and clear; this will encourage them to be open about their opinions and feelings
- Jointly decide on the best time to tell the child about a hospital visit, hospitalisation or treatment
- Involve only a few other staff so the parents do not feel overwhelmed by professionals
- Give medical information at a pace parents can cope with
- Name the disorder (whether or not the diagnosis is certain), treatment plan, prognosis and possible implications on the family, schooling, etc.
- Do not assume the parents know about the illness; they may only have hearsay or second-hand information
- It may be helpful to give parents written information, videos and names of parent support groups
- Be available to see parents on a regular basis, even if only for brief periods
- Act as facilitator to the parents and child adapting to the illness, especially chronic illness
- Discuss the importance of being honest with the child who may have overheard what was said between the doctor and the parents
- Parents of a dying child usually want to know how long the child will live and under what conditions the child will die. This information will help them to plan the remaining time and express their feelings
- Allow time for questions, concerns and opinions

should always be extended to both. Parents often feel blamed for anything that goes wrong with their child, so the doctor needs to choose words carefully when speaking to them. Staff should aim to give parents support, so that they can concentrate on helping to alleviate the children's anxiety. Parents often ask questions, especially at times of great distress, that may make the doctor feel uncomfortable. For example: 'How can you be so sure about the diagnosis of cancer? We would like further tests to be done, otherwise we shall go to another hospital'. Doctors sometimes respond inappropriately by giving reassurance, e.g. 'My daughter had the same and this is what happened and this is how she felt'.

In some cases, parents may neglect the child's needs. You will then need to make a referral to other professionals to ensure that the family receives support and that the child's development is being adequately nurtured and monitored. In other cases, some children might benefit by being referred to a psychotherapist, psychiatrist or psychologist who specialises in working with children; alternatively, the whole family might be referred to a family therapist. In making a referral to another professional, you always need to explain the reasons and allow time for the parents and the young person to ask questions, for example:

> "I feel that now that Jinny's asthma has stabilised she would benefit from spending some time talking to the child psychotherapist. She still seems to be rather upset and, as you said earlier, she has not been breathing well at night for the last few weeks."

In this case, the doctor explains why he thinks it would be helpful to refer to a therapist, providing a concrete reason derived from the parents' comments and his own observations of the child. The child also needs to be addressed, and the doctor should say to whom the child is being referred:

> "Jinny, I was just explaining to your parents that there is a woman I would like you to meet who knows a great deal about children and can help you."

If the child is ready to listen then one can take the conversation further to:

> "You could talk together about the bad dreams you've been having, and she could help you get rid of them. You could meet her tomorrow. How does that sound?"

For older children, there may be a need for more information, such as:

> "I would like to recommend a female psychologist, Dr H, who specialises in working with young people and asthma and she has also done a great deal of research on this topic."

Adolescents can be encouraged to make contact themselves with allied professionals. Often this gives them more power and more responsibility in their own treatment and welfare.

Professional colleagues

Child psychotherapists, child psychologists, child psychiatrists, family therapists, social workers and play workers are available to advise you on how best to work with a child or family. Also, they can be consulted about managing psychosomatic problems and the psychological effects of illness on children and families. Encourage the child to express feelings, verbally or through play: a fear may be irrational, but you should nevertheless encourage the child to express it so that you can offer reassurance or support.

Teachers

The child's teachers should be informed about his or her condition and what impact the illness might have on his or her family, school attendance and work. Teachers can be an important liaison because a child is often preoccupied about missing school and can be teased by other children about being ill or different. Provided there is consent from the child and parents, other school staff, who have significant support roles (such as catering supervisors or physical education teachers with the young person) can play a key role in maintaining as much normality as possible at school and supporting the young person's treatment.

Issues of confidentiality

Children and adolescents are often anxious that the information they disclose to the doctor will remain confidential. You need to reassure the child that you will not betray a confidence – otherwise, you could destroy the doctor–patient relationship. Young people who are ill can feel they have lost control over their body and environment, and this feeling of helplessness can be accentuated if they fear they have no control over which people know about their condition. When you feel that it is in the child's interests to disclose confidential information to his or her parents, you should explain to the child the reasons for your decision and the possible implications of disclosing the information.

Key points

- The doctor is the advocate for the young person, not for the parents or the hospital.
- Think of the young person as an individual who can provide important information on the diagnosis and treatment.
- Involve the young person in the treatment and explain each stage of the medical process.
- Relate to the young person according to his or her developmental age.
- Work together with the family, whenever necessary, as they can provide historical and developmental information on the young person which may be crucial.
- Work with other medical or non-medical professionals.

FURTHER READING

Brazelton TB 1976 Doctor and child. Delacorte Press, New York

Brazelton TB 1995 Behavioural assessment scale, 3rd edn. Mackeith Press, London

Brazelton TB 2006 Touchpoints: your child's emotional and behavioural development. Viking, New York

Brazelton TB, Sparrow JD 2002 Three to six. Da Capo Press, Cambridge, MA

Dowling E, Osborne E 1994 The family and the school: a joint systems approach to problems with children. Routledge, London

Garralda ME (ed.) 1993 Managing children with psychiatric problems. BMJ Publishing Group, London

REFERENCE

1. Winnicott DW 1992 Through paediatrics to psychoanalysis. Karnac, London

9

Communication with a patient's family

We are taught in medical school to think of the human body as a set of interrelated systems: change in one system can result in changes in another. For example, if you are late for an examination you will probably speed up your journey to the examination venue. As you run, your heart rate will increase, your breathing will become more rapid, you may begin to sweat, and so on. Similarly, a person's medical problems and illness have an impact on other systems that person inhabits, of which the family is probably the most significant. In the traditional medical model of diagnosis and treatment, we are taught to look for problems inside the person and then to target treatment exclusively at that person. However, we also know that the family can play an important role in the development and management of a person's illness.

As we have already seen, good medical care partly depends on our ability to communicate effectively with patients. In almost all cases, we also have to communicate with the patient's family and, occasionally, with other relatives or friends. Even if we do not have direct contact with anyone else, we may still need to consider their views and beliefs, as these may influence those of the patient. It is helpful to look at some of the issues that can arise when dealing with the patient's family, including: making an assessment of social support and of family beliefs, as they affect illness and treatment (e.g. non-compliance of treatment); and managing secrecy-related problems and confidential information (Fig. 9.1).

Some doctors find it a hindrance having to deal with the patient's family and relatives. It may demand more of their time and take them away from other duties. They may not see any value in involving the family in treatment and care. They also recognise that it may require special skills talking to a small group of people rather than an individual. Inevitably, difficulties arise where there are secrets between family members or where you have information that is confidential and the family demands to be told. It is not surprising that nurses sometimes feel that they are left on their own to look after the needs of the family.

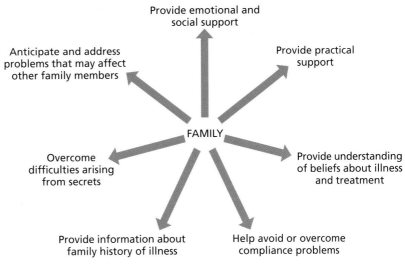

Fig. 9.1 How the family can help in diagnosis, treatment and care.

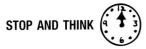

STOP AND THINK

If you or someone in your family has been ill, you probably had many questions about what would happen and what the outcome would be; we get anxious and annoyed without information or answers to questions. Consider how you would respond as a doctor to enquiries from a patient's relatives:

- *How do you know it is a relative you are talking to?*
- *How can you find out what the relative already knows?*
- *If the relative rings you, is there any information you would not give over the telephone?*
- *Is there anything you would tell a relative but not the patient (and vice versa)?*

At times of ill health, we look to others for support and may depend more on our close family and friends. But social support is not only concerned with practical problems, such as getting to and from the clinic or making sure that pets at home are fed while a person is in hospital. It also entails emotional support and comfort at a time when hope and self-confidence may wane. Studies have shown that social support can act as a buffer to psychological distress. There is also evidence that our bodies undergo physiological changes at stressful times such as the loss of partner, close friend or relative. The immune system is especially affected. Social support, therefore, can have an impact on both psychological and physical health. For this reason we must take care to help our patients sustain important relationships at times of illness, and to encourage them to draw support from others. We can assist in this task by talking about the family, asking questions about who the patient regards as close family and offering counsel where appropriate.

Observing the patient in context

You can usually make a preliminary assessment of a patient's support system even before asking about it directly. You can make the following observations:

- Has the patient come alone to see you?
- Has one relative come along, or is the whole family in the waiting area? What does this convey about how the patient and family view their illness and medical encounters?
- Has the patient been visited by anyone on the ward?
- Has the patient received cards, flowers or fruit?
- Has someone brought the patient personal items (e.g. toothbrush, hairbrush)?
- Does the patient mix with others on the ward, or remain apart?

Of course, this information does not reveal whether the patient prefers to draw on others for support or copes better without it. That can only be assessed by talking to the patient and asking about social support.

Identifying the patient's family

(p. 192)   **Exercise 8**   Although factual information may be needed about the patient's family to complete the background history, it is also important to ask about family and friends in order to identify those who are most likely to provide practical and emotional support (see Exercise 8). Take care not to make assumptions about who the patient would identify as 'family' (a patient could name a relative who is not a blood relation, or a partner of the same sex or a close friend). The following questions are useful:

"Whom do you regard as your close family?"

"Are you currently in a relationship with anyone?"

"Who else knows that you are here today?"

"You mentioned a partner: what about other family members such as brothers, sisters, parents?"

Once family members have been identified, or while gathering information about them, you could draw a family tree, sometimes known as a genogram or pedigree. This helps to organise and graphically represent information about relationships. Figure 9.2 shows the family tree of a patient with coronary heart disease: notice the familial pattern of the illness. A family tree includes details on gender, age and relationships, and it can also include an illness history. For a description of how to draw a family tree, see McGoldrick and Gerson.[1]

Having gathered details about the family, you can add the patient's views on the quality of these relationships and whether there are

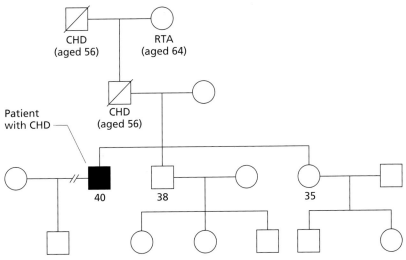

Fig. 9.2 A family tree. CHD, coronary heart disease; RTA, road traffic accident.

problems that may affect the patient and the patient's management. The following questions help to explore these issues:

> "Is there anyone who ought to know you are here today?"
>
> "Is there anyone whom you are afraid to tell?"
>
> "How often do you see (or have contact with) your parents?"
>
> "Whom could you ask for help with the shopping?"
>
> "You mentioned your sister: is there any reason you would not ask either of your brothers for help?"
>
> "How do you get along with your son-in-law?"
>
> "Who is most worried about you? How does that person show he or she is worried?"

Lastly, discuss more sensitive issues about the family, including changes in relationships and identifying the next of kin:

> "What ideas do other family members have about this illness or condition?"
>
> "How have things been with other family members since you learned the diagnosis?"
>
> "Who has been most supportive? Who the least?"
>
> "What support do you find the most helpful? Who best provides this?"
>
> "How do you think other family members see you managing?"
>
> "If something were to happen to you, whom would you like us to contact?"

The family's influence on care and treatment

A person who experiences ill health does not do so in a social vacuum. That person's concerns about the course and outcome of the illness are usually influenced by his or her previous experience of illness, by the illnesses of family and friends and by commonly held beliefs about the specific illness. For example, how someone might have contracted an illness can influence our ideas or prejudices about that person. Some people, including doctors, are prejudiced against people who smoke and who then need treatment for cardiac or respiratory problems. Similarly, public perceptions of infertile couples change when it is known that the same couple is also infected with HIV. Relatives of a homosexual man with HIV may see the illness as fair punishment for his sexuality. By way of contrast, a haemophiliac with HIV may receive sympathy from relatives who know his infection resulted from a blood transfusion rather than his own behaviour.

Beliefs about illness are also influenced by the nature of the condition – whether it is chronic, acute, relapsing, degenerative, infectious, and so on. The nature of the condition will determine the level of care, the length of time care is needed, and whether the onset of problems is likely to be sudden (and unpredicted) or gradual (and anticipated).

Sociologists have written about the 'sick role' in regard to the patient's relationships with professional carers and with relatives. We become more dependent on others when we are sick, and sickness can indirectly influence our relationships: relatives feel obliged to visit; doctors resist giving bad news for fear the patient's morale will be undermined; the liaison psychiatrist is called in when a patient becomes depressed, for example after a disagreement with a partner. The expression of a deceased relative ruling from the grave is also well known. Even relatives who are well can suffer as a result of illness in the family. For example, the brother of a boy with sickle-cell disease may play truant, shop-lift or bed-wet when the boy is admitted to hospital. The brother's behaviour may deflect others in the family from their own distress, or he may want to call attention to himself at a time when his brother receives more attention.

There is reciprocity in communication within a family. Relationships in every family, no matter how rigid or stuck they may appear, are dynamic and complex. At times of illness, in particular, each person's capacity to adapt is tested in response to new demands and circumstances. This is why family relationships are usually more tense and uncertain at these times. Our response (as doctors or as relatives) is either to withdraw or to become involved in a family crisis.

There may be times when it is important to address other family members' beliefs about, and experience of, illness. These can be explored by raising some of the following issues with either the patient or relatives or both:

"Has anyone else in the family suffered from a similar problem?"

"How have family members previously dealt with illness or death?"

"Who finds it most difficult to cope?"

"What changes have there been in family relationships since this medical problem first came to light?"

"Have there been any surprises with regard to how people have coped?"

"What ideas do family members have about this illness?"

"Whose views about health and treatment are most influential in your family?"

Treatment compliance and the role of family beliefs

It is important to address beliefs about illness and care, not only because this can help family members to cope and adjust to changing circumstances and relationships, but also because it may directly affect the patient's compliance with treatment. Because a doctor's knowledge of disease and treatment is assumed to be superior to the patient's, it is also assumed that the patient will automatically agree with the assessment and treatment plan. An impasse can arise, however, when a patient either subtly or directly rejects treatment but still maintains a relationship with health care providers. An example of this is a diabetic woman who will not alter her diet but regularly keeps clinic appointments. Many patients do not take the prescribed medication, while a proportion of those who do take it do not follow the instructions. A patient with depression may, for example, take antidepressants only when feeling depressed, rather than regularly, 'forgetting' that the treatment may take more than a week to have any effect.

An impasse is marked by a 'more-of-the-same' situation in which any advice by the doctor results in 'no change' in the patient (Fig. 9.3). The relationship between the doctor and patient is characterised by an increasingly desperate or authoritative doctor trying to convince an equally rigid patient to comply with treatment, to no avail. The result is a game without end, a source of frustration and annoyance to the doctor. The interaction becomes repetitive and rigid. It is sometimes maintained by misunderstandings on the part of the patient, or the doctor

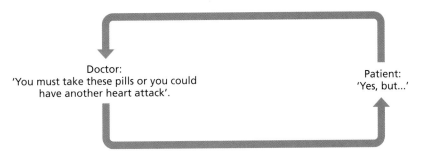

Doctor:
'You must take these pills or you could have another heart attack'.

Patient:
'Yes, but...'

Fig. 9.3 A non-compliant patient and an authoritarian doctor create an impasse.

not fully appreciating the patient's and relatives' views. There may be a belief that treatment only makes a problem worse ('I know someone who died while on those pills'), or that the patient should not trust medical advice ('My mother says you can cure that with plenty of garlic') or that treatment is not necessary or effective ('It's only a small bruise – it will soon go' or 'I'm 68 – I've had a good innings').

To avoid a potential impasse, you should check whether the patient understands the treatment goals and the role of medication. Give the patient the opportunity to ask questions or raise concerns. This also helps you to assess whether the patient is likely to follow the course of treatment. Lastly, ask if the relatives have any concerns, as you may need to take these into account when giving advice on treatment.

Working with couples

Surprisingly little research has been carried out into how adult couples cope with and adapt to illness. What we do know, however, is that the process of adaptation is influenced by a number of factors, including:

● the nature of the illness (e.g. acute, chronic, degenerative)
● the specific nature of the condition and how it affects the relationship (e.g. neurological, sexual)
● the onset (whether gradual or sudden) and the extent to which the couple could prepare for it
● the existing quality of their relationship
● previous personal and family experience of coping with illness
● the role of the person (i.e. primary bread-winner) in the relationship
● whether the illness is infectious and, therefore, whether both partners might be infected
● existing roles and relationships in the couple and family network, and the relationship between the couple and the wider kin network
● availability of support from relatives or other carers
● the developmental stage of the couple (i.e. whether they are newly weds or a couple facing old age)
● the psychological resilience of each individual.

When illness strikes a couple relationship, the effect may be either to destabilise the relationship or to create an even closer bond between partners. Sometimes it has the effect of doing both, although greater closeness is often preceded by a period of uncertainty and instability, both of which are normal. These fluctuating states occur as a result of primitive psychological feelings such as fear, anger, anticipatory loss, and fear of abandonment or loneliness. Partners may also sometimes have expectations of one another that are not met, giving rise to feelings of resentment. It is not surprising that tensions often rise when one's partner becomes unwell.

It is all too easy for the medical student or qualified doctor to feel caught in the middle of these complex relationship dynamics and feel 'pulled' to side with one or the other partner. For obvious reasons, this should be resisted, although it may be helpful to acknowledge some of the patterns of behaviour that you have identified. Take care to present these to the couple in a non-blaming way and pay specific attention to framing your thoughts or observations using conditional language. For example:

"Mrs Baldock, I wonder whether your husband's sort of...umm...annoyance with the nurses has something to do with him feeling uncertain as to how best to help you. Maybe he also wants to be a bit more 'hands-on' in taking care of you. He may need a bit more time to get used to what is happening to you and his own role in taking care of you. This may take a while as I understand that this is the first time you've been admitted to hospital."

or:

"Sometimes couples find it quite a challenge getting used to the changes that come about after treatment for this problem. One area that some couples find especially difficult adjusting to is the effect that the pills may have on sexual functioning. From what we have just been discussing, it may be that this is something that you are both having to adjust to, but I know from other patients we see here that this can cause distress and lead to more frequent rows. Some patients I have treated have told me how helpful it was seeing our counsellor who has a lot of experience in this area and with these problems. I was wondering whether you might want to think about meeting her and having an initial consultation to explore these issues?"

Responding to and managing the concerns and fears of relatives

Each family member will cope with and adjust to a relative's illness differently, depending on roles in the family. Some family members are better at providing practical rather than emotional support. Others are repelled by illness and either visit infrequently or only telephone to enquire about the patient's condition. By way of contrast, some families organise a 24-hour vigil and take it in turns to be with the patient at all times. Most children's hospitals and paediatric wards make provision for parents to stay overnight with their child. When relatives are anxious, they will naturally seek out a doctor to obtain information about diagnosis and the likely prognosis, among other issues. Sometimes, their enquiries can cause a number of difficulties:

- Relatives may approach different members of the health care team for information, and especially the most 'vulnerable', such as medical students and junior doctors. This happens especially when the senior doctors have not provided a clear account of the illness, prognosis and treatment. Medical students can be put in a difficult position in such cases because, although they may have the information, they may not be empowered to give it.

- Relatives may also seek out different doctors caring for the patient in a drive to 'get the truth', or a word of hope in a seemingly hopeless situation. The dilemma for you is whether to give false reassurance (and possibly give them temporary relief) or repeat what they have been told (and run the risk that they may continue to search for more palatable news).
- A relative may attempt to control the dissemination of information to others (including the patient), claiming that it would hurt the person to know. Although protecting someone may be viewed as caring, it also gives rise to secrecy and alliances, and adds complexity to relationships. Moreover, it raises questions about the limits of confidentiality and whose interests are best being served.

The ways in which the family responds to illness can also create problems in communication and management. Relatives can:

- not recognise (deny) that a problem exists and so not take appropriate action. For example, the parents of a teenage girl who has been dieting and lost a great deal of weight may dismiss suggestions that she is becoming anorexic. They may fail to confront her about it and resist seeking professional help.
- believe all problems can be solved and take action when it is not necessary or appropriate. For example, the parents of a child involved in a serious accident are told that the child is brain-dead and can only survive with the aid of a ventilator. They insist on ventilating the child against professional advice.
- mishandle a problem by applying the wrong solution. For example, a man becomes overstressed at work and gradually develops irritable-bowel syndrome. His wife encourages him to drink alcohol to calm his nerves. This exacerbates his symptoms, and the attempted solution becomes a new problem as the patient also develops liver disease.

Skill and tact are necessary to manage each of these difficult situations. The doctor must take care not to undermine the confidence and competence of the relatives. At the same time, you may have to give advice and new ideas that may be strange to the patient and family, regardless of their background and nationality. Our task as doctors is to give explanations and not expect people to adjust to them immediately. Rather than blame the patient and relatives for misunderstanding or for creating an impasse, you should first consider whether you have created the problem yourself.

Guidelines for dealing with a patient's family

The following guidelines can help us to look after the patient's relatives and reduce the chance of difficulties when dealing with them:

1. Acknowledge their support.
2. Speak to them and give them time to raise issues or concerns.

3. Where possible, provide them with a room where they can be alone.
4. Identify a key worker (e.g. nurse or doctor) whom they can contact. Tell them how they will be contacted if the patient's health deteriorates.
5. Before giving information to relatives, first give it to the patient and check whether you have the patient's permission to discuss it with others.
6. Ask the patient who in the family can be given what information.
7. Write up a summary in the notes of important discussions with relatives so that your colleagues know what has been said to them.
8. Where secrets arise, talk to colleagues about how you might deal with them. As a general rule, remember that the patient decides what information, if any, can be given to others. When in doubt, tell the relatives to ask the patient if you are not free to discuss something with them.
9. If the patient is very unwell, encourage relatives to make frequent, but short visits.
10. Do not examine the patient (unless a child) in front of relatives.
11. Do not carry out procedures (such as taking blood) in front of relatives. Ask them to leave the room.
12. Do not discuss family issues in ward rounds.

Dealing with problems arising from secrets

The Hippocratic oath states that the doctor's duty is not to disclose information to anyone but the patient in the course of treatment. This privilege, however, is not without exception or limitation, particularly where harm to others outweighs confidentiality, such as in the case of a notifiable infectious disease. More common are problems arising from secrets between family members, such as relatives not wanting to tell the patient the diagnosis, or vice versa. There is a difference between secrets and confidential information. Secrecy means keeping information from others, whereas confidential information is a shared secret, perhaps between the patient and professional carers. Problems usually arise when those who feel it is their right to know suspect that certain information has been suppressed. There are three major kinds of secret:

1. *Individual secrets*: one person keeps something private from others, e.g. a man is worried about a chest infection and has recently lost weight, but resists going to his GP for fear he will be admitted to hospital for tests.
2. *Internal secrets*: two people share information not disclosed to others, e.g. a patient is treated by his GP for a sexually transmitted disease; this is not disclosed to the patient's wife, who is also one of the GP's patients.
3. *Shared secrets*: information is known within a circle of relationships but is withheld from others, e.g. the close family of a young patient decide not to tell other relatives that the child was born with a congenital abnormality.

Boundaries and alliances between people can be created, strengthened or destroyed by secrets. They can generate anxiety within relationships. Keeping a secret usually has both positive and negative implications. A secret may bring into focus themes associated with exclusion and dishonesty. At the same time, almost all secrets serve to protect someone from something. Doctors are not excluded from the effects of secrets, which can create considerable stress and lead to a feeling of being immobilised by the patient. At times, we may consider it our task to take sides, to advise patients or to expose the secret. Occasionally, we help to generate secrets. After a patient has been given the results of a laboratory test or a diagnosis, some doctors prescribe secrecy by suggesting that the patient not tell the result to anyone, for fear of strong emotional reactions or rejection. Doctors can take a number of steps in order to minimise the sometimes harmful effects or stress experienced on account of secrecy (Table 9.1). Some of the steps are illustrated in Case example 9.1.

Table 9.1 Managing secrecy-related problems

- Establish whether a secret exists. Clarify your role in relation to it (e.g. are you being asked to share confidential information?)
- Do legal or ethical concerns apply? (e.g. Hippocratic oath, public health laws, duty to warn others of a threat to life)
- Clarify the dilemmas involved in keeping the secret and discuss them within the clinical team and, where relevant, with the patient. Sometimes a general discussion is sufficient to resolve the problem
- Weigh the advantages and disadvantages of keeping the secret. Discuss the range of possible outcomes with the patient
- What prevents disclosure is the fear of its consequences. Ask hypothetical questions to help people imagine the consequences, e.g. 'What might be your son's reaction if he knew that you may need surgery?'
- Without disclosing confidential information to relatives, you can still discuss hypothetical possibilities, e.g. 'Obviously, I can't give you that information. You will need to ask Mr Corney. But if he were to have cancer, what would that mean to you? And what does his reluctance to talk about his illness say to you?'
- Establish with the patient who can be told what about the patient's condition. This will reduce pressure on you and your colleagues. Talk with the patient if relatives continue to demand information. Reassure the patient that you will not breach confidentiality, but that you may ask relatives to consult the patient when they next approach you

---

Case example 9.1

Patient unwilling to tell husband of her hospital admission

Mrs Potts, aged 69, saw her GP because she had been having dizzy spells and chest pains. She had not told her 70-year-old husband about the symptoms or her visit to the GP. The doctor was concerned about her blood pressure and wanted to admit her to hospital for some tests.

MRS POTTS: *Oh, I couldn't possibly do that! I couldn't tell my husband. And anyway, who'd look after him?*

DR CHURCH: *I can understand your concerns. If he knew that you had come here today, what do you think he would say?*

MRS POTTS: *He'd be so worried. You know Gerald – he doesn't like it when anyone is sick, and he hates hospitals. Maybe I can tell him I'm going up north for a few days to see my sister.*

DR CHURCH: *What do you think would most worry him?*

MRS POTTS [TEARFUL]: *If something happened to me. I've always thought it would be me looking after him, not the other way around. He wouldn't manage on his own.*

DR CHURCH: *Yes, you've been together, what – nearly 45 years? It's hard to think about the changes that happen as we get older, especially after such a long marriage. But let's not jump to conclusions. After all, this is for tests. If you were in Gerald's shoes, would you want to know?*

MRS POTTS: *I suppose so.*

DR CHURCH: *So how might you tell him?*

MRS POTTS: *I don't think I could face it. You can see, I break down just like that, and he'd get very upset and worried. Can you tell him?*

DR CHURCH: *Yes, I can. If you'd like, I'll come round at the end of the surgery today. But it would be helpful if you think about what you will say to him. It sounds as if the worries you have for one another may need to be more openly discussed between you. You might also think about what you will say to your sister and daughter.*

MRS POTTS: *One step at a time please, doctor!*

(p. 193) **Exercise 9** Secrecy-related problems are a recurrent feature of clinical management and can arise between doctors and patients, patients and their families and between health care professionals themselves. Often, the limits of confidentiality are tested. If you explain to the patient the dilemmas that secrets can cause, you can remove a source of stress from the relationship. You will also give the patient the responsibility for resolving problems. Asking future-oriented and hypothetical questions is a non-confrontational device that will help some patients to consider ideas they might otherwise fear to address. Learning how to manage secrets can also lead to more open communication, not only between the doctor and patient, but also between the patient and relatives. This helps to involve others in practical and emotional care and support, and to address problems with treatment compliance (see Exercise 9).

Key points

- Illness not only has an impact on individuals, but also affects the close family and relatives.
- Family members usually provide practical and emotional support, so it is important to address their personal concerns and their role in care-giving.

- Do not make assumptions about who the patient defines as 'family'.
- Drawing a family tree provides a graphic representation of relationships and clues to patterns of illness between generations.
- The patient's family can influence treatment compliance.
- Secrets can create an impasse in care and interfere with personal and professional relationships.
- The use of hypothetical and future-oriented questions helps to overcome an impasse.

FURTHER READING

Bor R, Gill S, Miller R et al 2008 Counselling in health care settings. Palgrave McMillan, Basingstoke

Launer J 2002 Narrative based primary care. Radcliffe Publishing, Oxford

REFERENCE

1. McGoldrick M, Gerson R 1985 Genograms in family assessment. WW Norton, New York

10

Mistakes, complaints and litigation

"To err is human; to forgive, divine."

We all make mistakes; Alexander Pope expressed this in the above quotation that also recognises the difficulty of dealing with mistakes and their consequences. Some mistakes are trivial, have no significant consequences and pass unnoticed. Some have serious consequences and may threaten the lives of patients under our care. They may lead to complaints from patients or even to law suits against the doctors involved.

How should we react to our own mistakes and those of others? How should we deal with patients who complain about the treatment they receive? The way we communicate in such situations is vitally important and may greatly affect the outcome.

Making mistakes in everyday life

Admitting our mistakes is difficult. Yet recognising when we have made a mistake and reflecting on why it happened often provide an excellent learning opportunity. Before considering errors in medical practice, we need to think about how we deal with the mistakes we make in everyday life.

  STOP AND THINK *First of all, think about a mistake you made recently in your daily life, for example when you were driving, or something you said or did that was hurtful to others. Was there an identifiable cause? How did you feel? What did you do? What did you say to the other person?*

Depending on the nature of the mistake you might have:

- passed it off as 'one of those things' and did nothing more about it
- felt very guilty
- blamed it rightly or wrongly on someone or something else
- admitted your mistake and apologised to the other person
- tried to analyse why you made the mistake – was it something you did wrong or was it due to a problem in the system?

- reflected on your analysis and resolved to avoid making the same mistake again.

STOP AND THINK *Now think about an occasion when you were affected by someone else's mistake. What did you expect of them? Go over the above list again. How did you react to their mistake?*

There is no doubt that it is often difficult to admit that we have made a mistake and it often takes courage to acknowledge it both to ourself and even more so to the other person. Here is an example in a medical setting for you to think about.

STOP AND THINK *You are on a ward round with your consultant who is known to be demanding and expects high standards from students and colleagues. She asks you to present the patient who was admitted the previous night having had a myocardial infarction. You have interviewed and examined the patient but realise during the ward round that you have forgotten to measure his blood pressure, which is a key aspect of the examination. The consultant asks you: 'What was the patient's blood pressure on admission?' What would you say?*

The options would be to be honest and admit that you had not measured it or to make up the blood pressure measurement. This would be unacceptable and could harm the patient – honesty is always the best policy.

Mistakes in medical practice

Studies in the UK,[1] USA and Australia have shown that a significant number of patients suffer an 'adverse event' during their stay in hospital. An adverse event is defined as 'an unintended injury caused by medical management rather than the disease process'. In the pilot study in the UK, which was based on a retrospective review of over 1000 hospital notes, the authors found that 10.8% of patients suffered an adverse event that could be attributed to some aspect of their care. A third of these patients suffered disability or died.

How often do doctors make mistakes? In a questionnaire survey of junior doctors they were asked about the frequency of making mistakes.[2] The authors of the report classified mistakes into minor, moderate and major.

- Minor mistakes were defined as actions that did not result in the patient suffering pain or discomfort – but corrective action should have been taken.
- Moderate mistakes resulted in the patient suffering pain, discomfort or temporary or permanent disability, but the patient's life had not been in danger.
- Major mistakes resulted in a patient's death or his or her life having been in danger.

Of the doctors who responded, 77% said that they had made a minor mistake during the previous month, 24% had made a moderate mistake during the previous 2 months and 16% reported having made a major mistake during the previous year.

Causes of medical mistakes

So mistakes are relatively common and are rarely the fault of one person. Consider the following case and think about the factors that contributed to the mistake.

Case example 1

A fatal mistake

Robin Smith, aged 17 years, had leukaemia and was admitted to hospital because he had relapsed and was found to have cerebral involvement. Dr Jones, a junior doctor, was asked to perform a lumbar puncture and inject methotrexate intrathecally. He felt tired and anxious but was relieved when he carried out the lumbar puncture successfully. He reached for the vial of methotrexate from the trolley and injected it easily. Ten minutes later Mr Smith had a convulsion and died. Dr Jones looked at the vial for the first time: it said 'for intravenous injection only'.

There are a number of possible contributing factors to this error that had such disastrous consequences. The key mistake was that Dr Jones did not check the contents of the vial before injecting it into Mr Smith's spine. Why might this have happened?

- He might have done it because he felt tired and stressed and couldn't think straight.
- He was inexperienced and had never even seen the procedure carried out.
- He could have forgotten or had never been taught that it is essential to check a drug before administering it.
- The vials of methotrexate for intravenous and intrathecal use looked very similar and the nurse had taken the first one to hand and had not checked it.
- The nurse who was helping him was called away as he was carrying out the procedure.

If you think about these possible contributing factors, you may see that they fall into two distinct groups: first, those relating to Dr Jones, and second, those relating to the system and not associated with him. These include the similarity of the two vials, the failure of the nurse to check them, and the fact that Dr Jones had been working long hours and was, therefore, more error-prone.

What implications does this have for the management and prevention of medical errors? First, it is usually inappropriate to blame one person. Errors are usually multifactorial and invariably involve aspects of how tasks within the health care system are organised and carried out. Hospitals are complex organisations in which risks to safety of both patients and staff abound. The emphasis is now on managing that risk:

first, by looking carefully at procedures to identify potential risks and dealing with them, and second, by learning from errors that do occur by reporting and analysing adverse incidents and near misses. In this way adverse incidents can be prevented and patient safety improved. For example, in the UK intrathecal chemotherapy must now be formally checked by a nurse, a pharmacist and a physician before it is given to a patient.[3]

What should you do when you have made a mistake?

This clearly depends on the circumstances and consequences of the mistake. Some guidelines are given in Table 10.1.

Table 10.1 What to do if you make a mistake

This depends on the circumstances and the nature and consequences of the mistake, but here are some general guidelines

Do:
- be honest – admit it to yourself and tell a senior colleague
- be prepared to discuss it with the patient
- listen to the patient's or relative's concerns and demonstrate that you are listening
- apologise – this is not necessarily an admission of guilt
- make a record in the patient's notes – a factual statement of what happened
- analyse with the help of others why the error occurred
- seek help if you feel burdened by what has happened

Don't:
- become defensive
- accept or assign blame
- criticise others
- 'go it alone', particularly if the consequences of the mistake have been serious. Students and junior doctors should not be expected to handle situations such as that described in Case example 1

Should you tell the patient even if he or she has not suffered any ill effects? A recent study found that the majority of patients questioned would want to be told.[3] However, this is a difficult thing to do. Consider what you would do in the following example.

Case example 2

Admitting your mistake to a patient

The registrar on your firm asks you to take blood from Mr Thomas who has severe rheumatoid arthritis. You have great trouble getting the blood from one of the veins in his forearm and he complains of pain. You put the blood into the bottle and are about to send it to the laboratory when you realise that you have used the wrong bottle. The blood test is important and you return to Mr Thomas to take another sample. What would you say to him?

STUDENT: *I am very sorry, Mr Thomas, but I am afraid that I used the wrong sort of blood bottle. It's very important that we send your blood to the laboratory today. I realise that you had some pain when I took the last one. How would you feel about me taking another sample?*

MR THOMAS: *Well, it was a bit uncomfortable but if you've got to do it then you've got to do it so go ahead.*

This is another example of an error that might have been prevented if the system of blood collection had been designed differently. It is possible that the blood bottles were very similar in appearance and this increased the chance of the student making a mistake and choosing the wrong one. This might have been avoided if the bottles were of different colours.

Recording errors

It is essential to make an accurate record of what has happened in the patient's notes. Remember that what you write should be:

● accurate and clear
● avoiding ambiguous abbreviations
● legible
● dated, with your name in capital letters, and signed.

Consequences of medical errors

In Case examples 1 and 2 the consequences of the mistakes that were made were very different. In the first one Robin Smith, a previously fit young man, died. In the second Mr Thomas, an elderly man with a chronic illness, suffered discomfort but no long-lasting effects.

This illustrates the range of consequences of medical mistakes for patients. The responses of patients or their relatives also range from accepting an explanation and taking it no further to making a formal complaint or taking legal action against the doctor and hospital.

Complaints

The number of complaints by patients is increasing. This increase is a reflection of patients' increased expectations of health care professionals and the increasing culture of consumerism within the health service. Patients have a right to complain if they feel that they have received an inadequate service. This might be the result of a diagnostic error, a mistake in their treatment, poor communication or the unprofessional attitudes of staff.

Some examples of poor communication that may lead to complaints are shown in Table 10.2. A patient's complaint may be fully justified, for

Table 10.2 Examples of communication problems that may lead to patients complaining

- They think that they have not been given enough information about their treatment and therefore have not given fully informed consent
- They believe that they have been treated in an insensitive manner
- They feel that they have been ignored

example the patient may have been kept waiting for an unacceptably long time in the outpatient clinic with no explanation or apology. It is important to remember that sometimes a patient's complaint may reflect his or her anxiety or anger about an unrelated matter and you should deal with this as discussed in Chapter 11.

Very often the motive for a patient or relative making a complaint is to seek an explanation for what went wrong and to prevent the same thing happening to someone else.

Dealing with complaints

The key thing is the way in which complaints are handled; some guidelines are given in Table 10.3.

Investigation of complaints should be seen as an opportunity to improve the quality of services that a hospital provides for its patients. Moreover, the early and sympathetic handling of a patient's complaint is less likely to leave the patient feeling aggrieved and resorting to legal action.

Table 10.3 Dos and don'ts for handling a complaint

Do:
- be sympathetic – even if you do not think that the complaint is justified
- apologise when appropriate
- give a full verbal explanation to those involved
- seek advice from a senior member of staff
- keep good notes
- maintain confidentiality

Don't:
- avoid the complainant
- get angry or defensive
- try to cover up – always be honest about what happened
- tamper with the notes
- criticise a colleague

Preventing complaints

The majority of complaints arise because of communication problems rather than negligence, and are best dealt with in a sympathetic, sensitive manner. There is evidence that developing and maintaining good communication skills decrease the likelihood of a doctor receiving a complaint.[3] A recent study in Canada has shown a link between the communication skills scores of doctors in an examination they took soon after graduation and the number of subsequent complaints made against them.[4]

Litigation

Unfortunately it is becoming more common for patients to take legal action against doctors. This is distressing for the patient and stressful for all involved in the patient's care. A study of patients and relatives in the UK[5] found that they took legal action after an incident because they wanted to:

- know why and how the injury had happened
- prevent a similar injury to other patients
- see staff disciplined and held to account
- gain compensation.

Very often the decision to take legal action after an incident is strongly influenced by the way in which the incident is handled by staff. The patients and relatives interviewed in the study described above complained that they had not been given an adequate explanation of what had occurred, there had been no apology and they were often treated as if they were neurotic.

Once again, the way in which a doctor communicates with the patient is important. A study in the USA found that 1% of hospital patients had suffered significant injury due to medical negligence, but that less than 2% of these had brought a malpractice claim against the doctor involved.[6] The authors compared the communication skills of the doctors who had claims against them with those who had no such claims. They found that the 'no claims doctors':

- used more humour in the consultation
- used more facilitation statements like, 'What do you think the problem is?' and 'Go on...'
- told the patient what the doctor was going to do, for example: 'I just want to ask a few questions about your work' and 'Now I would like to examine your back'.

The message from this study is that developing good communication skills improves patient care and also reduces the chance of litigation.

Key points

■ Mistakes in clinical practice are inevitable.

■ Mistakes are usually due to a combination of people factors and systems factors.

■ If you think you have made a mistake and feel upset, be sure to seek help from a colleague.

■ Blaming someone for a mistake is usually inappropriate – the emphasis is on establishing a blame-free culture in which we can admit mistakes and learn from them.

■ We can learn from mistakes by analysing what went wrong and learning how similar mistakes may be avoided in future.

■ When mistakes happen, communicating sensitively and effectively with patients, their relatives and with colleagues helps all those involved to deal with the situation.

■ How you communicate with patients and their relatives influences their decision about making a complaint or taking legal action.

REFERENCES

1. Vincent C, Neale G, Woloshynowych M 2001 Adverse events in British hospitals: retrospective record review. British Medical Journal 322: 517–519

2. Baldwin PJ, Dodd M, Wrate RM 1998 Junior doctors making mistakes. Lancet 351: 804 (letter)

3. Cave J, Dacre J 2008 Dealing with complaints. British Medical Journal 336: 326–328

4. Tamblyn R, Abrahamowicz M, Dauphinee D et al 2007 Physician scores on a national skills examination as predictors of complaints to medical regulatory authorities. Journal of the American Medical Association 298: 993–1001

5. Vincent C, Young A, Phillips A 1994 Why do patients sue doctors? A study of patients and relatives taking legal action. Lancet 343: 1609–1613

6. Levinson W, Roter DL, Mullooly JP 1997 Physician–patient communication. The relationship with malpractice claims among primary care physicians and surgeons. Journal of the American Medical Association 277: 533–559

11

Challenging consultations: special problems in doctor–patient communication

Geraldine Blache and Robert Bor

In this chapter we shall explore some of the more challenging aspects of meetings with patients. In particular, we shall look at ways of communicating effectively with patients who:

- are withdrawn and appear difficult to engage in conversation
- are anxious
- are angry and aggressive
- have hearing and/or speech problems
- are knowledgeable or even experts about their medical condition.

The chapter includes a case study of a challenging consultation that illustrates how good communication skills are both a diagnostic and a therapeutic tool. The case example also illustrates how important it is to develop empathy with a patient.

The uncommunicative patient

Communicating with people who do not themselves want to communicate is not a problem confined to the medical consultation. We have all encountered this kind of situation at some time or other. Maybe you are or have been uncommunicative yourself.

What are the kinds of things that make us more or less willing to communicate? How will we know if someone is being uncommunicative in this particular setting, or if this is just his or her usual manner? Is it merely because the person's style of communication is different to ours that we find it a challenge? Think about recent social occasions where you have wanted to get to know people unknown to you.

For some people, starting a conversation with complete strangers is an effortless activity, while for others it is a daunting challenge. Many factors affect our ability to talk easily with people we do not know well, including:

- Our personality or general disposition – are we outgoing, gregarious, shy, self-conscious, empathic?
- Our previous experiences of meeting people – what has been our experience of approaching strangers? Have we been rebuffed, encouraged, overwhelmed?
- Our state of mind – are we angry, anxious, depressed, hung-over?
- The reputation of the other person – what have we heard about that individual? What preconceptions do we have?
- The physical appearance of the other person – is he or she scruffy, smart, attractive or physically unattractive?
- The other person's behaviour – is he or she aggressive or overpowering, does the person fidget or fuss?
- The context and the geography of the meeting – is it welcoming, friendly, noisy, private, too secluded? Are the chairs too close, or too far apart? Is there something of importance at stake?

These factors, and others, influence communication even before a word is spoken and should help us to understand why a patient appears reluctant to talk. The patient may be:

- naturally shy and reserved
- embarrassed about some aspect of his or her problem or of demonstrating ignorance of it; the individual may be taken aback by your questions (e.g. about sexuality, bowel habits, income or social circumstances)
- feeling sad or depressed
- in pain
- wanting to obstruct the consultation for reasons known only to that person.

So you first need to consider why the patient appears to be uncommunicative:

- Is the layout of the consulting room inhibiting the patient? Are you sitting too close or too far away? Could the individual have doubts about the privacy of the consultation?
- Has some aspect of your behaviour disturbed or inhibited the patient?
- Does the patient's body language indicate how he or she is feeling? Is the person obviously in pain? Does he or she look anxious, shy, embarrassed, sad, depressed?

Remember too the cultural differences in relation to communication and, in particular, to notions of space between people, eye contact and notions of modesty.

Notions of appropriate behaviour

The depressed patient

What do we mean by 'normal' behaviour and how do our beliefs about normality affect our communication? At the break-up of a relationship, or after failing an exam, we are likely to feel low. These powerful emotions can be frightening to us and possibly to those around us. However, they do not, of themselves, necessarily indicate clinical depression (for which specialist help should be sought) but rather a migration along a spectrum of 'normality' in response to challenging events. In experiencing such feelings we hopefully gain insight into the sense of helplessness such events can bring.

Depression can give us a sense of helplessness, and ordinary daily activities become an intolerable drudge as concentration fades and unhappy thoughts intrude on our seemingly fragile lives.

In the normal course of events, these feelings (despite our perceptions at the time) are transient episodes in an otherwise stable life: our ability to cope overcomes the grief and sadness. We grow through our experience, and in consequence develop a better understanding of the depression of others.

If we sensitively listen to and question a patient who seems depressed, we can place that person's sadness within a spectrum of emotions which are normal or abnormal for that particular patient. Perhaps the patient feels he or she is expected to display sadness over the death of a loved one, even if this is not how that person is experiencing the loss. As you make your judgements about the patient's psychological state you might also consider whether what you take to be a problem for your patient is merely a reflection of your own, probably different, assumptions about life and how it should be lived. If the patient does not socialise in the way you think he or she should or, for example, attend the local pensioners' luncheon club, or parent and toddler group, think about whose problem this is. Patients are individuals with individual needs and emotional responses. What may be considered normal for ourselves may, for someone else, be quite the opposite.

STOP AND THINK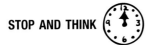

- *Is it a problem for the patient that he or she is feeling sad?*
- *Is the behaviour or emotional response normal for this particular patient?*
- *Is the patient trying to live up to your expectations of his or her reactions or behaviour?*
- *Whose problem is it?*
- *Patients are individuals with individual needs and responses; normality is subjective.*

Whatever the cause of the patient appearing to be withdrawn and uncommunicative, following some simple guidelines will help you to engage the patient in the consultation (Table 11.1).

Table 11.1 Guidelines for helping the uncommunicative patient

- Be prepared to spend time over the consultation
- Find ways of overcoming boredom, frustration and anger in yourself
- Observe the patient carefully: be alert and respond to the patient's verbal and non-verbal cues
- Show empathy by your own body language (e.g. lean forward and maintain eye contact)
- Explain the purpose of the interview: why you want the information
- Use facilitatory language, e.g. 'I can see that you're finding it difficult to talk about this'
- Use more closed questions than open questions, where this seems appropriate

---

The anxious patient

Anxiety is, of course, a normal and sometimes healthy response to life events. Here is a situation you might have experienced already.

Lorna is a final-year medical student now well past the stage of feeling the 'adrenaline rush' of meeting her first patients. She remembers the ordeal well enough though:

LORNA: *It was just awful. We were told to go and clerk a patient – no support, no offers of a helping hand, no explanations as to how it would feel to do this – to take a history and examine a patient. What should I say? 'Here I am, I know I'm the same age as your daughter – your granddaughter, for heaven's sake – but I've just got to ask you to undress and to answer all these really intimate questions.'*

QUESTIONER: *How did you do it then?*

LORNA: *Well, I'd get to the door of the ward. I'd stand there, seeing the patient in bed, knowing what I had to do. Then, before I knew it, I was just soaked – everything, all of me, I was sweating from head to toe. I'd have to go off and have a shower!*

QUESTIONER: *And did you come back?*

LORNA: *Oh yes. I got through the door after a few attempts. By the time I was able to walk through the door and go up to him in bed you could actually see my heart leaping out of my chest. My face went from scarlet to ashen and I developed a tremor ready to compete with any patient with Parkinson's disease on a ward round!*

Lorna's experience will ring true for many of us. What she was describing was a 'normal' anxiety attack which, thankfully for Lorna, was reasonably short-lived and something that she can now look back on and laugh. Lorna's ability to do this, however, is due to her understanding of what was happening to her at the time.

Drawing on your own experience of anxiety can help you to empathise with an anxious patient and create a more holistic picture of the patient and his or her illness. As with the uncommunicative patient, it is important to recognise when a patient is anxious. The person may:

- show the physical signs of anxiety: sweating, flushing, trembling, fidgeting
- speak rapidly in an uncontrolled way
- seem to be making excessive demands on you, particularly for reassurance.

You should also try to understand why the patient is anxious:

- It may be the patient's usual behaviour: the person may have an anxious personality, or be suffering from a chronic anxiety state.
- It may be the patient's response to his or her illness and to receiving medical care. Most of us feel some degree of anxiety in these circumstances: fear of dependence, of what might be wrong with us, of the future.
- The patient may feel anxious about other problems.

In the consultation, it is important to help patients to feel less anxious (Table 11.2).

Table 11.2 Guidelines for helping the anxious patient

- Be calm and prepared to spend time with the patient
- Explain that most patients feel some anxiety and that this is appropriate
- If the patient is talking too much, try to keep the patient to the point by summarising what the person has told you and explaining what further information you need and why you need it
- Be specific about what you may want the patient to do during and after the consultation
- If the patient presses you for the cause of his or her symptoms and seeks reassurance, explain that you are a student and refer the patient to his or her own doctor

---

The angry, aggressive patient

We prefer to think of medical settings as a refuge from the real world, which can be violent, unpredictable and uncaring. In practice, however, this is sometimes far from the truth. An increasing number of health care staff are physically attacked or verbally abused by patients. This is not confined to accident and emergency services, even though this is often portrayed in television soap dramas. Violence may be directed at us because the patient is angry with something we may have done (or forgotten to do), such as having kept a patient waiting. Tempers may also flare because the patient feels frightened and helpless, or has received bad news. Whatever the cause, your communication skills will be extensively tested and, in all likelihood, the outcome – whether someone is assaulted or the threat abates – will largely depend on what you do and say.

The most important tasks are verbally to break the cycle of anger and aggression, and reduce the threat of harm to everyone, including the patient. You should not contradict the patient or behave in a threatening way; usually, this will only make the problem worse. Your priority should be to create a calm atmosphere so that normal activities can proceed without a threat of violence. Prevention is best:

- Do not become combative.
- Be 'street-wise': do not work alone in settings where there is a potential threat.
- Think ahead. Some doctors scan their consulting rooms and remove from easy reach objects which may, in extreme circumstances, be used by a violent patient against them.
- Memorise the telephone number of the security guards, or at least always keep the number by the telephone.

As a matter of good housekeeping, ensure that the team in which you are working has regular drills to ensure that safety alarms work and everyone knows the correct procedure in case of violent attack. Prevention is better than cure so consider a range of get-out sentences for whenever you feel uncomfortable – perhaps saying that a significant page of the notes is missing or that you need to ask your colleague about something. Hopefully you will never have to use any of these but knowing that you have planned for such eventualities will give you an added confidence which will be reflected in your consultation.

The best advice when confronted with a threatening patient is to stop and think before acting. You should follow steps that will help to de-escalate the threat of violence (Table 11.3).

Table 11.3 Guidelines for dealing with the angry or aggressive patient

- Is the patient agitated, restless or ready to explode? What does the patient's behaviour communicate to you?
- Show willingness to talk and listen. Acknowledge the patient's anger or annoyance. Never redefine the person's behaviour as fear or anxiety, even if the patient seems to manifest these feelings
- Keep a safe distance: neither too close, nor too far away
- Do not: interrupt the patient's outburst; caution a swearing person about his or her choice of words; threaten the patient in any way
- Ask open rather than closed questions. Encourage the person to talk: talking is preferable to violent behaviour
- Do not make agreements or promises that cannot be kept; be reasonable and honest
- Help the patient to feel he or she has choices: people are most often aggressive when they feel they have few or no choices
- Do not talk to the patient from behind: this can be threatening and unnerving. Also, do not attempt to touch the patient: any movement could seem threatening. On the other hand, do not block the person's path: ensure the patient has an escape route
- Do not take personal offence at what might be said; this could make you aggressive or defensive and so escalate violence
- Never let down your guard until the incident is over. Fatigue, or a sense that the argument is ending, could lead you to take risks and so start up the problem again
- If security staff are summoned, try to supervise their actions so that you maintain some control over the situation

Signs of distress

Learn to recognise signs of anger or distress in order to defuse a situation before it gets out of hand:

- speech (becoming louder and quicker or becoming quiet)
- facial expression (changing, flushed, loss of eye contact)
- manner (impatience or non-compliance)
- body language (closing in, or sudden or expansive movements).

Both you and your patient may experience one or more of the above signs. Unless you recognise them and take steps to deal with the emotions, it is possible for the consultation to disintegrate into a spiralling decline with neither doctor nor patient gaining from the experience. Do not deny reality, no matter how painful. Learn to confront it and open up communication.

Developing awareness

Acknowledging our limitations and being prepared to challenge them can occasionally help us to understand our patients as well as ourselves. We can learn and practise skills to help us cope with unpleasant emotions we may encounter during a consultation. Anger and violence are as much a part of grieving as are acceptance or sadness. To deny or dismiss anger prematurely can delay a necessary healing process. Maintaining the fine line between staying with the patient at this time and accepting gratuitous abuse is something that will only come with time. Paramount is your personal safety so take this opportunity to learn from, as well as with, your more experienced colleagues.

How you communicate with your patients, relatives or colleagues under stressful conditions will help determine the outcome of the consultation. Remember the skills above and practise them. Be alert to the setting of a consultation and to non-verbal feedback. Above all, try to put yourself in the patient's position. For example, think about how you might respond to bad news, to feelings of worthlessness or despair, or to an instance of medical negligence (or what might appear to be medical negligence). Moreover, remember that people taken out of their normal environment and put into stressful situations may well behave out of character.

Patients with speech and/or hearing problems

Probably very few of your colleagues in medical school and hospital – particularly doctors and nurses – suffer from a disability that affects how they communicate. Our experience of people with a disability most likely derives from members of our own family or from the patients we meet. A significant part of medical practice involves the diagnosis and treatment of congenital or acquired disabilities, and the counselling of patients and their families to adapt to the consequent unwelcome circumstances. Diagnosis, treatment and counselling are especially challenging when the patient's hearing and speech are impaired.

People of any age can be affected by speech and hearing problems and for this reason we should not make assumptions about who may be affected. Nonetheless, we know from clinical practice that many doctors cope with these problems better if the patient is young rather than elderly. It can feel awkward trying to communicate with an adult who has difficulty hearing or speaking, whereas with a child, we typically revert to signs, symbols and activities similar to play (e.g. pictures, pointing, monosyllables, and so on).

The process of ageing often leads to speech and hearing difficulties. Reaction time slows, concentration decreases and serious medical events, such as a stroke, lead to loss of ability to communicate effectively. Other family members may themselves suffer; we often hear in consultation with a partner or spouse that the patient has become intolerable since becoming demented or suffering the stroke, or becoming deaf. Many ageing processes or medical events are irreversible, but we should not dismiss them. The increased prevalence of mostly untreatable speech, visual, auditory and motor problems among the elderly should not imply that treatment and care should be all but abandoned. Instead, communication, in whatever form, should take on a new level of importance. The patient can become depressed if socially isolated and neglected. Furthermore, other problems that are potentially treatable – such as insomnia, constipation or a tremor, among others – could be overlooked.

The process of denial is similar with children. Parents of children with communication problems may believe that the child is slower than others but will later catch up. They may thus not immediately recognise the problem. Difficulties with speech may be put down to shyness. Concomitant problems with social behaviour may signal auditory, visual and speech problems. These may be overlooked by people who know the child well. Teachers, the school nurse and parents of other children may be the first to point out that the child does not seem to hear properly, is inattentive or listens selectively. Others may compensate for the child's inadequacies by completing half-finished sentences or by infantalising the child.

Doctors are at a disadvantage with a patient much younger or much older than themselves. To a child, we may represent an authority figure and, therefore, an unsympathetic adult. Moreover, we are seen as having the capacity to inflict pain (through injections, treatment, and so on). Children may feel intimidated, constrained or anxious in our presence. To older patients, we may represent highly technical and alienating medical practice. Some older patients may be fatalistic, having grown up in an era in which there were less effective methods of diagnosis and treatment. A proportion will have survived local catastrophes, wars and other forms of adversity. It is not surprising, therefore, that difficulty in communication is exacerbated by an apparent lack of understanding or empathy.

Much research has been carried out into social attitudes to people who have difficulty communicating. Social distance increases when someone is hard of hearing, deaf, has a speech impediment or is unable to communicate predictably and clearly. This leads to feelings of embarrassment, annoyance, impatience and frustration. Some people with a disability avoid social contact. In turn, we learn little about how to improve how we communicate and may misinterpret signs: someone who keeps to himself may be labelled a recluse, antisocial, crazy or stubborn. There are two problems that we must, therefore, overcome: how to avoid situations in which attempts at communicating may be challenging or embarrassing (Fig. 11.1), and how to improve our repertoire of communication skills with patients (Fig. 11.2) who have a range of disabilities. Table 11.4 shows what we should not do when we speak to someone with difficulties in communicating.

STOP AND THINK

- *Whose responsibility is it in a medical consultation to ensure that there is effective communication – the doctor's or the patient's? Why?*
- *What can you do to improve communication if the person you are talking to: (a) is hard of hearing? (b) quickly forgets what has already been said? and (c) cannot express him- or herself clearly?*
- *What is your own response to someone with one of these disabilities? How do you think this has come about? Is there anything you can do to improve how you would communicate?*

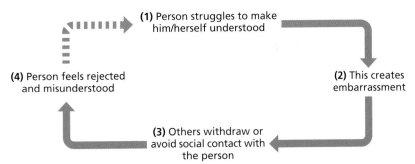

Fig. 11.1 Communication problems which may be experienced by people with a disability.

(1) Person struggles to make him/herself understood

(2) This creates embarrassment

(3) Others withdraw or avoid social contact with the person

(4) Person feels rejected and misunderstood

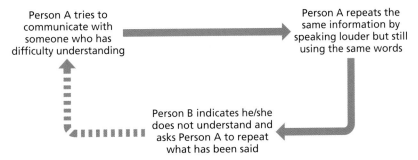

Person A tries to communicate with someone who has difficulty understanding

Person A repeats the same information by speaking louder but still using the same words

Person B indicates he/she does not understand and asks Person A to repeat what has been said

Fig. 11.2 Improving communication with patients who have a range of disabilities.

Table 11.4 How not to respond to a person with communication difficulties

Don't

- Repair language (to someone who is stuttering): 'What you are trying to say is: Will I go home this week? The answer is yes'
- Tell the person what to do and think: 'If you don't say anything, we must assume you don't want to go on the day trip. So you'll have to stay behind and sit in the day centre'
- Patronise: 'Leave her alone; she doesn't understand what we're saying. You'll only upset her'
- Speak louder: there is a tendency to increase the volume of speech rather than use different words, believing that the louder we speak, the more easily the other person will understand us
- Use another person as conduit for communicating (in front of the patient): 'What is he saying? Can you understand?' [under your breath and exasperated]: 'I give up!'
- Become impatient and angry: 'Look, I've got a busy clinic. If there's something else, speak to one of the nurses'
- Offer meaningless reassurance (after incomprehensible sounds from a patient): 'Don't worry, we'll take care of everything for you'

Remember the basic axioms of communication:[1]

- One cannot not communicate
- Communication is usually both verbal and non-verbal
- Every communication has an implied statement about (or definition of) the relationship with another person or audience.

Hints and examples for talking to a patient with a communication disability

Do not ignore the person

Avoidance can lead to new problems, such as the patient feeling unimportant. Learn about the disability by talking about it with the patient: is the condition auditory or verbal, or is it related to a cognitive, learning or organic problem?

Dr Lategan:	*I'm afraid I don't quite follow what you are saying. Could you repeat that for me?*
Mr Walsh:	*It's b . . . b . . . b . . . b . . . been th . . . th . . . th . . .*
Dr Lategan:	*Are you trying to tell me it's been on your skin for a long time or a short time?*
Mr Walsh:	*Long.*
Dr Lategan:	*By the way, do you often stutter, or is it just with someone you don't know very well?*
Mr Walsh:	*Someone I . . . I . . . I . . . don't know.*
Dr Lategan:	*That's all right. Take your time. I'll ask if I don't get it.*

Do not make assumptions about what the patient is trying to say

If necessary, establish a different method of communicating that allows the patient, for example, to point at a word or picture. Some patients who have great difficulty hearing or expressing themselves can be asked to respond with a 'yes' or 'no' to a series of questions (verbal or written) that explore a problem.

DR ROSS:	*Mrs Smith, I'm going to ask you some questions to help me to understand what is going on here. All you have to do is answer 'yes' or 'no'. If you prefer, you can nod or shake your head. Is that OK?*
MRS SMITH:	*Yes.*
DR ROSS:	*Did anyone bring you to casualty?*
MRS SMITH:	*Yes.*
DR ROSS:	*Was it your husband?*
MRS SMITH:	*No.*
DR ROSS:	*A relative?*
MRS SMITH:	*No.*
DR ROSS:	*A friend?*
MRS SMITH:	*Yes.*
DR ROSS:	*Did your friend see what happened in the kitchen?*
MRS SMITH:	*Mmmm.*
DR ROSS:	*Yes?*
MRS SMITH:	*Mmmm.*
DR ROSS:	*No?*
MRS SMITH:	*Mmmm.*
DR ROSS:	*Maybe?*
MRS SMITH:	*Yes.*
DR ROSS:	*Do you remember where on your head you were hit?*
MRS SMITH:	*No.*
DR ROSS:	*Does it hurt at the back of your head?*
MRS SMITH:	*Yes [and so on].*

Use other forms of communication

These include sign language, pointing to written words or symbols and writing. Ensure that both you and the patient understand the meaning of signs and symbols.

Use an interpreter (or third party)

Using an interpreter or third party when the patient has difficulty with speaking, hearing or understanding is controversial. Doctors sometimes complain that interpreters summarise what is said and thus alter the meaning of the communication. Furthermore, problems relating to confidentiality arise, particularly with regard to personal information. Where potentially embarrassing information needs to be discussed, ask the interpreter to leave and use another approach with the patient (such as those described above). If you feel that the interpreter is editing too much of what is said, ask the person to translate exactly what has been said.

MR DLAMINI: *[long explanation in Zulu]*

INTERPRETER: *He says he gets dizzy.*

DR CLARKE: *Now I want you to translate exactly what he said. It is important I understand everything.*

INTERPRETER: *Sometimes there are voices. They tell him to fetch his cattle and bring them to London because they will be stolen. Then his mouth gets dry and he gets dizzy.*

DR CLARKE: *Now ask Mr Dlamini if these voices are inside his head, or does someone talk to him? [and so on]*

Check the patient's understanding

Ask the patient to repeat what has been said, or to summarise the conversation. This prevents misunderstandings and helps to assess whether the patient has short-term memory problems or difficulty retaining information.

DR JOHNS: *I just want to check that you understand which pills to take and when.*

MR FINE: *The yellow one in the morning, and the others – Oh, I think – no – maybe . . .*

DR JOHNS: *That's OK. Now, what do you usually do if you need to remember something important?*

MR FINE: *It's best if I write it down. Then I won't forget.*

DR JOHNS: *Here's some paper. The yellow one once a day before breakfast; the large round one three times a day after meals; and these small ones when you need one for sleeping.*

MR FINE: *I'll tell my wife too. She's good at reminding me.*

If the patient has dementia

Practical considerations need to be made for the care of patients with dementia. Memory problems are most common. For this reason the patient may need to be reminded about appointments and routines. This also reinforces social contact, which may be important to someone who is becoming disoriented. Carers may themselves need positive encouragement, as they can become easily frustrated in their efforts to communicate with the patient.

Keep talking to the patient

If a patient is unconscious, unable to speak or is being ventilated in intensive care, it is still possible that the patient's hearing is intact. A calm and familiar voice can reassure a patient who feels isolated or abandoned. In some situations, it may be possible to set up a system of communication in which you talk to the patient, and he or she responds by squeezing your hand. A 'yes' can be one squeeze and a 'no' two squeezes. The pattern of communication follows that described in the point *Do not make assumptions about what the patient is trying to say*, above.

Accept help from parents or carers

In addition to using some of these approaches yourself when communicating with children who have auditory, visual and speech difficulties, you can use the parent's or carer's knowledge of the child to help you. They can act as translators or interpreters. It is sometimes helpful to use a favoured animal noise to communicate. You may need considerable patience until the child learns to feel sufficiently comfortable with you before you attempt to talk about medical issues.

Case example 11.1

A challenging consultation – whose challenge?

Mrs Celia Lazio is a teacher aged 42 years, married to Tom and with two children, aged 16 and 10 years. She is a serious person but also enjoys a good laugh. She enjoys her work and combines a full-time career with the needs of a growing family. Since her husband was made redundant last year after a motorbike accident rendered him unable to work, she is the main wage-earner. They make do and are not overly worried about their financial state.

Eight years ago, Mrs Lazio noticed a worsening of her chronic 'bad back'. Infrequent 'attacks' had recently increased in intensity and her ability to carry out many routine tasks declined. Pain and worries about the future frequently interrupted her sleep, which left her exhausted and unable to cope with the day ahead. Her GP referred her to a rheumatologist.

At the clinic

Having enjoyed nothing but good health in the past, Mrs Lazio found the clinic a frightening experience. The rheumatologist, Dr Morley, was friendly but failed to put her at ease. The consultation focused on her pain: its type, intensity, duration and what helped it. The physical examination was painful and distressing, confirming Celia's worst fears about the extent of her reduced flexibility. Her pain and fears affected her behaviour. The consultation concluded in this way:

DR MORLEY: *I'm giving you a sick note to cover you for 2 weeks while we investigate further.*

MRS LAZIO: *I don't need a sick note, thanks. I'm not off work.*

DR MORLEY: *Well, you should be, my dear! Do you realise what you are doing to yourself going to work in that state?*

Mrs Lazio:	*Well, I've managed this far, thanks all the same.*
Dr Morley:	*Four weeks! I'm changing it to 4 weeks and make sure you stick to it.*

Mrs Lazio broke down in tears. Dr Morley, not unsympathetic but concerned about his waiting patients, showed her the door and warned her that if she ignored his advice, she would exacerbate her complaint.

What was happening in this consultation? Developing effective communication skills takes time and the ability to reflect on practice. Let us look again at the same consultation but this time, consider:

- Was the patient in pain, or depressed?
- What does she make of her 'back pain'?
- What do 'being ill' and being off sick mean to her?
- Who is Celia Lazio?
- Is this a caring doctor?
- What are they communicating to each other, and with what consequences?

Here is their consultation again, but this time, the rationale behind the responses is given:

Dr Morley:	*I'm giving you a sick note to cover you for 2 weeks while we investigate further.*
Thinks:	*This woman is obviously in pain and needs rest. Best to let the inflammation subside while tests are carried out.*
Mrs Lazio:	*I don't need a sick note, thanks. I'm not off work.*
Thinks:	*Aghast at thought of time off. Confirmation that she is ill; worries about keeping job; too busy to be ill; what would happen to her family if she got sick?*
Dr Morley:	*Well, you should be, my dear! Do you realise what you are doing to yourself going to work in that state?*
Thinks:	*Clinical worries about exacerbating condition: doing herself more harm; has range of possible diagnoses in mind but doesn't share them for fear of upsetting Mrs Lazio; will tell her when he has test results.*
Mrs Lazio:	*Well, I've managed this far, thanks all the same.*
Thinks:	*I can't deal with this right now – blanking off – doesn't want to hear any more.*
Dr Morley:	*Four weeks! I'm changing it to 4 weeks and make sure you stick to it.*
Thinks:	*I am acting in her best interests: she finds it difficult to take time out. I'll make the decision for her. She is obviously depressed: just look at her. She's waiting for me to take the decision and needs someone to be firm.*

Mrs Lazio broke down in tears. The pain was unbearable now, as was this pompous and patronising doctor who didn't understand anything about her, or how she had coped over the years. She had managed before and certainly could do so again without being off work for 4 weeks.

The rheumatologist was also angry: 'Why did these people come to him for advice and then not take it?' His professional opinion was being ignored and he felt personally affronted. Before showing her out and recommending again that she follow his advice unless she wanted to end up 'not being able to walk at all', he inserted in her notes: 'Patient very depressed'. A follow-up appointment was made for 1 month. The sick certificate read 'spondylitis?'.

STOP AND THINK

- *Questions relating to the nature and source of pain are an essential part of making an accurate diagnosis, but so, too, are questions about the experience of pain – on the patient's life and self-image, for example.*
- *Physical examination is an essential part of diagnostic procedure, but it may be the first time a patient realises the extent or severity of his or her condition.*
- *The consultation (interview and examination) can be tiring and sometimes traumatic. We need to consider what effect this has on the way a patient responds to questions, suggestions and treatment regimes.*
- *Even if the consultation is neither tiring nor traumatic, we need to consider the implications of seeing someone removed from his or her normal setting and routine (e.g. symptoms may be exacerbated or lessened by this).*
- *Was the sick note the best way for the patient to discover what she took to be her 'diagnosis'? What is the significance of the question mark – for the doctor and for the patient?*
- *What does it feel like for the doctor to have his professional opinion queried or ignored?*
- *Decisions about clinical management cannot be taken without regard to personal, social or emotional circumstances.*

In this consultation, both parties were talking but were they communicating effectively? Dr Morley:

- collected various diagnostic clues from the patient
- had nowhere to go with these, apart from making a provisional diagnosis, but even this might not be confirmed by the test results
- did not encourage patient involvement
- did not inspire confidence in his patient
- had little chance of compliance with any suggested treatment, so the benefit of a diagnosis is short-lived.

In his own way, Dr Morley is a caring doctor who thought he was doing right by Mrs Lazio by taking decisions out of her hands: he deemed her to be emotionally and physically unable to take the decisions herself.

On the other hand, Mrs Lazio was:

- feeling less and less in control of what was happening
- picking up clues from the consultation that led her to take an even more pessimistic view of her health problems
- scared and vulnerable
- coping by pretending none of this was happening at one level, while at the same time recognising that it was all too real.

(p.193) **Exercise 10** Dr Morley assumed Mrs Lazio was depressed because of her responses. However, because he kept these observations to himself, he had no way to check with her if she was indeed depressed and, if so, what they might do about it. Instead, his views were confirmed by her tearful outburst, rather than by anything she said. At this point, he chose to relieve her of further distress by deciding that what she needed was a break from her work.

The follow-up visit

In the month since her last visit, Mrs Lazio did take time off work. In the event, the pain, made worse by the examination, was bad enough to prevent her from returning to work even if she had wanted to. She spent much of her time in bed, frightened to move too much in case her condition worsened. The effect of this was to make her sleeping problems even worse and her back was a great deal more painful and stiff.

On her follow-up visit, she saw a different doctor. He introduced himself as Dr Peter Parker and explained that he was the senior registrar:

DR PARKER: *That seemed to be hard work getting up from the chair and walking in here?*
(Acknowledging her pain: professional validation.)

MRS LAZIO: *Yeah.*
DR PARKER: *So, how has it been?*
MRS LAZIO: *What? Me, or my back?*
DR PARKER: *Do you see them as different then?*
(Questioning and probing.)

MRS LAZIO: *[silent for a while] Yes, I suppose I do. I often find myself saying I'm OK but my back isn't. Funny that, isn't it! [pause] I don't know.*
DR PARKER: *Know what?*
(Mirroring, reflecting.)

MRS LAZIO: *I just don't know. That's the trouble. I just don't know – anything. My mind has gone to pot over the last few weeks. I feel so out of touch with reality.*
DR PARKER: *What is reality for you then?*
(Using patient's vocabulary.)

MRS LAZIO: *Well, you know. I don't know what's happening at work. I'm not sure I know what's going on at home either!*
DR PARKER: *What has been happening?*
(Still open; not reframing in order to fit his own agenda.)

MRS LAZIO: *Well, Tom, that's my husband, he's been looking after things. Doing the shopping, clearing up, making sure the kids are OK.*

DR PARKER: *And that's a problem?!*

(Use of humour, at the right level and right time.)

MRS LAZIO [HESITATES]: *No. No, of course it's not.*

DR PARKER: *Does he often help around the house like that?*

(Is this normal for this particular family?)

MRS LAZIO: *No, never, not unless I ask. He'll always do it if I ask. Willingly that is, he's not a complainer [pause]. He did used to help. We always used to split the chores – he always did less of course, being a man! No, I liked to do it and he liked to do his bit, but then when he got made redundant, it stopped.*

DR PARKER: *Why was that, do you think?*

(Not making his own assumptions or, where he does, he checks them out, investigating how insightful the patient is.)

MRS LAZIO: *Funny you should say that because I did a lot of thinking about that myself while I was laid up. I think he stopped because he didn't want to be seen as the househusband. His ego took a bit of a bruising after the accident. Not just losing his job – although that was bad enough. It was more to do with him having to stop training for a while. He's got a good body, he likes to keep in trim – but after the accident, he put on a bit of weight and it was a while before he got back into training again. I'm not sure how we got on to this!*

DR PARKER: *Well, let's think about it, how did you?*

(Using 'you' instead of 'we' encourages the patient to think about why she has mentioned these things in the consultation today; she associates them with her pain.)

Having helped Mrs Lazio to make some connections between her home life and her physical and psychological health, Dr Parker enquired about her pain and how she dealt with it:

DR PARKER: *So, you've told me about your pain: where it is and when you get it.*

(Making clear that he remembers, and that this is not the information he is seeking now.)

Tell me about how you cope with it. It's obviously very painful, I can see that.

(Reaffirming and acknowledging continued pain.)

MRS LAZIO: *It's funny, but hearing you say that – well, I don't think any-*
              one said that to me before. Not that I want them to know how
              bad it is, of course.
DR PARKER: *Why's that, then?*
MRS LAZIO: *Well, no one likes an old crock sitting in the corner, do they?*
(Cultural norms of expressing pain: hiding it, 'stiff upper lip', the
shame of illness ('why me?'), disablement, vulnerability, loss of
libido, physically draining, mentally disabling, depressing, disorien-
tating, drug reactions.)

              Besides which, if they knew at work what pain I'm really in,
              they would probably insist on me going off sick again.

(Repeated anxiety about losing job: is she happy in her work?
How does she benefit from it (apart from a salary)? What part does
her job play in her self-image? How does she feel about being the
main wage-earner?)

DR PARKER: *Sounds like there's lots of things going on there, Celia. Shall*
              we start to unpick some of them?

Dr Parker uses his counselling skills without turning the consultation
into a counselling session. In order to treat her condition effectively,
he needs to understand the context in which the condition occurred,
is reinforced, and in which he hopes she will recover. His 'unpicking'
the various aspects will involve acknowledging, then putting aside,
some issues, as well as pursuing those which directly affect the patient's
physical state.

Summary of Mrs Lazio's case

During the next couple of consultations, Dr Parker and Mrs Lazio
continued their exploration of the significance of her illness and how
this might be affecting her experience of pain. Mrs Lazio was able to discuss issues with this doctor that she had been unable to discuss with the
first rheumatologist or her GP. Given time, she was able to discover for
herself that, although the prospect of a disabling condition had made
her depressed and anxious, what she was experiencing could not be
attributed to the condition alone. Until she met Dr Parker, she had been
accustomed to 'sweep things under the carpet', emotionally and physically. Her inability to do this now in a practical sense (e.g. to leave the
housework to her husband) meant that she was also unable to sweep
aside the increasing load of anxieties lurking in her mind.

Given her success with the rheumatologist, Mrs Lazio saw her GP
again, and arrangements were made for both her and her husband to
attend a short course of counselling. Celia knows more about her

condition now and realises that her worst fears were based on outdated information. She recently attended a special pain clinic where both she and Tom learned more about the nature of pain and how it can be managed. The course was a real success and a small group of participants decided to carry on meeting at the end of it as a way of offering each other support – and to have a bit of a laugh!

What might have happened had she continued to see the consultant, Dr Morley? It is likely that the next consultation would have resulted in a referral to a psychiatrist. The referral in itself might not have been inappropriate, but the senior registrar, Dr Parker, had the skills to address her needs within the time-constrained routine follow-up visits.

Severe pain and chronic or incurable illness imply a patient confronting much more than a diagnosis. Doctors need to understand this so that they can offer patients the care and treatment appropriate to their individual needs.

We now turn our attention to another challenging consultation: where patients already have information about their condition before they see the doctor. Some may even be well informed and this may add a potentially complex layer to the doctor–patient relationship.

The informed patient

The traditional approach to the doctor–patient relationship assigned expertise to the doctor. Consequently, patients were almost wholly dependent on the doctor for all their information about the nature, treatment and prognosis of their condition. This hierarchically arranged doctor–patient relationship also had the effect of defining communication patterns between doctor and patient. For example, some patients might have felt too intimidated to ask questions of their doctor, while some doctors might have opted not to share too much information with their patient as there was little risk of the patient challenging the doctor. Medical students often feel at a disadvantage when talking to some patients because patients may know more about their condition than the student. The best advice we can offer is to acknowledge that this is the case and to ask patients confidently to teach you about their experience. For example:

> STUDENT: *I realise that many people have already asked you to describe the symptoms you have been experiencing, but it would be very helpful for me to hear about these and for you to tell me about your treatment as well and how you have been coping with this condition.*

Developments in information technology and the changing expectations of the doctor–patient consultation have come to challenge the notion that the doctor is always the expert. The most obvious changes that have dramatically increased the amount of information that patients may have include:

- access to the internet
- the influence of patient support and advocacy groups
- increased awareness of health-related issues (e.g. newspaper columns and magazine features).

Indirectly, other events and developments have also affected the balance in the doctor–patient relationship. The increased threat of litigation and the appalling abuse of trust within the doctor–patient relationship (e.g. Dr Harold Shipman's actions, as well as those of some other doctors) have contributed to the emergence of a more equally balanced relationship as well as increased collaboration between doctors and their patients. As we discussed in Chapter 2, medical consultations have recently become much more patient-centred.

Informed patients present a challenge to doctors who are used to, and feel more comfortable with, being in control of most aspects of the professional relationship. Patients who are knowledgeable about their condition, treatment, rights or any combination of these may not easily accept that all expertise has been ascribed to the doctor and, indeed, may have very different needs and expectations of the consultation. It is vital that these needs and expectations are considered and addressed, otherwise one of two (or even both) unwelcome outcomes is inevitable:

1. In seeking to assert his or her authority and set the agenda for the consultation, the doctor will, in all likelihood, become argumentative or combative with the patient. The more the patient does not feel listened to, the more the tension in the relationship will escalate. This in itself can have further consequences and, in some cases, the patient may become threatening or resort to physical violence in order to assert his or her views. A more likely outcome will be that the patient submits a formal complaint about the doctor and the case is yet another statistic of poor professional communication.
2. The doctor will cease to be useful to the patient. This could lead to decreased contact, loss of influence and even loss of status in the patient's eyes.

In the modern era, doctors need to adapt their style of communication and consultation to take into account the informed patient. For some, this may be a bold step to take as it requires a higher level of professionalism and a willingness to work more collaboratively with the patient. Developing a more positive connection and collaborative working relationship with patients requires a subtle shift in your verbal and non-verbal communication skills in the context of a consultation. The first task is to assess what it is that the patient is really seeking from you. To assume that all patients require the same help or information from their doctor is a gross error. It is helpful to start all consultations with:

DOCTOR: *How best can I be of help to you today?*

Notice how the doctor has deliberately not asked, 'What is the problem?', as this would assume that the patient has sought help for a particular problem. It would also inadvertently place the doctor in the expert/problem-solver mode. The more open-ended opening line described above also allows the patient to set the agenda. In the case of a well-informed patient, he or she might respond as follows:

PATIENT: *Well, doctor, I have read that lipodystrophy is a possible side-effect of this medication and because I also have hepatitis C, it would be unwise to change to the other medication because of the effect this could have on my liver. But I'm not happy with the effect this has had on my physical appearance and I wondered what you would advise?*

In this scenario, the patient conveys not only that he has some understanding of his condition and the associated problems with treatment, but that he faces a potentially difficult choice and has sought the opinion of his doctor. Notice too how the patient has defined the problem and has been clear about his goal for the consultation. Assuming that the doctor knows something about the particular patient and his medical condition, but is not an expert on that problem, the doctor might feel that he or she does not know much more than the patient, particularly where it comes to advising about a treatment dilemma of this nature. It is essential that you be honest about what you know and do not know in these and similar circumstances. If you try to conceal your ignorance you may appear to be inept, uncertain or foolish. Where you do not know the best answer to a question, it is crucial that you convey professionalism and confidence in not having the information or answer that is being sought. In other words, the doctor can still convey skill, sensitivity and professionalism in explaining that he or she does not know the answer. For example:

DOCTOR: *That's an interesting question. I can see that there is a dilemma here and, to be truthful, I do not currently have sufficient information myself to give you the best advice. Would it be helpful if I looked this up for you in the medical literature and had a chat with a specialist colleague who works in the hospital and I could then get back to you?*

Notice in this short excerpt that the doctor first acknowledges the patient's question and dilemma and conveys that he or she has at least listened to the specific concern. Stating that he or she does not currently have sufficient information also suggests that this can change; relevant information can be sought and this may change how the doctor feels about being able to respond to the question. Finally, the doctor tells the patient what he might do to inform himself so that he is aware of the doctor's next actions with regard to his enquiry. The doctor also poses this as a question to the patient, thereby checking whether the patient would indeed find this helpful. This is an example of a collaborative relationship with a patient. The doctor in this context is a further resource to the informed patient and not having the answer to a question does not diminish the patient's perception of the doctor or confidence in the doctor. Some doctors who work in a more consultative way have found that they feel less pressured and responsible for making decisions as they share some of the responsibility for decision-making with patients. Being seen to be a full-time expert is ultimately a burden and can be stressful.

Access to information about health, illness and treatments has changed the doctor–patient relationship. We cannot simply hide behind old knowledge or ignore the fact that some patients know more than we do about their condition. However, instead of feeling threatened or unnerved by informed patients, we should adapt our consultations accordingly. In the first instance, we should seek to understand what it is that the patient specifically wants from us at that moment. In so doing, we establish the basis for a more collaborative professional relationship with our patients.

Key points

- When communicating with patients who seem withdrawn, anxious or angry, try to understand the underlying reasons for their behaviour and adapt your style to facilitate communication.
- Notions of 'appropriateness' or 'normality' are not fixed: they depend on the individual culture and life experiences of both doctor and patient.
- When confronted by an angry patient, do not do anything that may escalate the threat of violence.
- Act conservatively: try to prevent situations from becoming worse by being attentive and concerned.
- Do not avoid patients with a disability, especially those whose hearing, speech and memory are impaired. Use both verbal and non-verbal forms of communication creatively.
- Use an interpreter where necessary. It can be helpful and important to ask the interpreter to translate exactly what the patient has said.
- Check that the patient has understood what has been said.
- Allow time for communicating with patients who have the difficulties discussed in this chapter.
- Many patients are well informed about their condition and this demands a more collaborative style of consultation.

FURTHER READING

Bor R, Gill S, Miller R et al 2008 Counselling in health care settings. Palgrave, London

Breakwell G 1997 Coping with aggressive behaviour. BPS Books, Leicester

MacDonald E 2004 Difficult conversations in medicine. Oxford University Press, Oxford

Silverman J, Kutz S, Draper J 2005 Skills for communicating with patients, 2nd edn. Radcliffe Publishing, Oxford

REFERENCE

1. Watzlawick P, Beavin J, Jackson D 1967 Pragmatics of human communication. WW Norton, New York

12

Communicating with patients and colleagues: learning more about how personal issues affect professional relationships

That's the reason they're called lessons,' the Gryphon remarked: 'because they lessen from day to day' (Alice in Wonderland, *Chapter 9*).

Even though he was not referring to teaching in medical school, Lewis Carroll had a point. Most students at some stage question the relevance of parts of their course, and the way they are taught, to the medical career they have chosen. This is especially true of students in their preclinical years, but it also applies to those on the wards and in GPs' surgeries. One student recently complained:

"We are taught in medical school to wear gloves when taking blood from patients to protect us from blood-borne infections such as HIV and hepatitis, yet the specialist registrars sometimes don't wear them on this ward. Is there a risk? Who is right?"

Another student suggested there was little incentive to read up on a patient's condition before a teaching session:

"The consultant makes a point of trying to show up someone in the firm. No matter how much we've prepared, the consultant always says, 'Yes, but...'. No praise. No encouragement. It turns one off studying."

Of course we hope that most of your course is stimulating and challenging, and that it will provide opportunities to discuss with fellow students (as well as teachers and consultants) confusing and frustrating issues such as those described above. This chapter addresses some processes in communication that may arise for medical students. It aims to develop a wider understanding of communication in context, and of roles and relationships.

Personal development

Throughout our lives we encounter change. Personal development is punctuated by a series of life stages – birth, infancy, childhood, adolescence and so on – and our ability to communicate progresses with each stage. We learn to communicate through social interaction and, primarily, through family life. Social development, including the acquisition and development of language, is intricately related to family development, roles, relationships and transgenerational patterns. How you relate to people and communicate is influenced to a large extent by the interactive patterns in your own family. Many factors are relevant in this regard, including:

- Your position in the family (as an only child, the eldest sibling, the youngest child, for example)
- Family rules or beliefs about communication (e.g. 'One has to be an adult to be taken seriously', 'Children should be seen and not heard')
- Transgenerational patterns (e.g. 'Only the views of male members are regarded', 'Opinions count only when you have left home', 'No one speaks about feelings because it is viewed as a sign of weakness')
- The structure of the family (e.g. 'There were so many of us at home that it was difficult to be heard')
- Legacies from past family events ('Nobody dared question my father ever again after I had a terrible row with him', 'Only my mother spoke openly about feelings after my brother died in an accident, and a few years ago she became clinically depressed. Now there's an idea in the family that a stiff upper lip in the face of adversity can prevent one from going mad').

STOP AND THINK 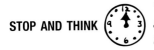 *You may recall that Chapter 9 covered communication skills with the patient's family and described how drawing a family tree could be useful in a medical consultation. Draw your own family tree and include a minimum of three generations.*

- *Can you use the family tree to gain an understanding of patterns of relationships in your family?*
- *What do you know about patterns of illness in your family?*
- *Does your family tree reveal any clues as to why you chose to study medicine?*

Indicators of how you communicate

Confidence in relationships and how you communicate with family and friends also influences interaction with peers, teachers and patients. Although you might not have been asked about this topic directly in your interview for medical school, in all likelihood it would have been part of the assessment of your suitability for training. The interviewers would have noted some of the following factors about how you communicate:

- fluency
- tone
- pace

- ability to understand English (and/or the language of the country)
- if your interactive style reflects rigidity or flexibility in thought processes
- congruence and relevance of content and process
- if you can put others at ease in an interview
- emotional maturity; ability to deal with challenging situations
- possibly, also, whether you have a sense of humour.

Context is crucial in understanding communication: people's expectations are defined by the context in which they communicate. Your behaviour and language probably differ depending on your situation: a conversation with friends in the pub will be more relaxed and friendly than a conversation during an interview.

But context is only one marker of communication. Others include personal and social development, which implies the changes in how we communicate and what is implied by our communications as we move through different stages of life. The transition from school to university is for many young people the most significant stage in the process of leaving home. It marks two major changes. The first is in oneself: one becomes more separate and autonomous. The second is in relation to one's family: the family structure may not change, but patterns in relationships may alter as new roles are defined; meanwhile, new relationships are established and different patterns of relating emerge. But the leaving-home transition does not signal the end of changes in relationships. You will probably be able to identify some of the changes between when you first started at medical school (say in your late teens) and when you qualify in your mid-20s. Perhaps you have gained confidence, acquired new friendships, ended a romantic relationship and started to plan ahead for your career in medicine.

Changes in how you relate to peers and friends may also signal a change in how you communicate with patients and colleagues, and vice versa. Perhaps some ideas in this book, together with training in communication skills on your course, may also influence you. Moreover, patterns of communication develop as a result of events in your personal life. For example, you may find it difficult to give bad news to a patient if someone in your own family has recently died. Medical complications caused by a patient's lifestyle (such as alcohol abuse) may trigger your own frustration and resentment if you grew up disapproving of excess drinking. How we feel about our patients in a given situation can cause us to communicate with them in ways that may be unhelpful. At times, you may 'block' the patient by changing the topic of conversation and sidestep the issues or concerns the patient wants to address. Similarly, you may offer reassurance or give advice to a patient at a time when listening is called for, or perhaps ignore the emotional concerns of the patient and instead just focus on the physical aspects of the problem. Most of us have at some point been guilty of giving false reassurance or simply 'jollying' a friend, relative or patient along because we did not have not the time or capacity to deal with more complex emotional issues (Table 12.1). It is normal inadvertently to 'block' the patient once in a while, especially when you are feeling stressed. However, this behaviour could suggest a more worrying problem about one's communication patterns or ability to deal with expressions of emotion if this becomes a pattern in how you relate to patients or, indeed, others.

Table 12.1 may help you identify situations when there is an impasse in communication with a patient, or when the management of a patient's problem becomes excessively stressful. Of course, because we relate differently to different people does not necessarily mean we have one of the problems listed in Table 12.1. We may have a problem, however, if we repeatedly relate to a patient in one of the ways listed, and so establish an unfortunate pattern.

Table 12.1 Patterns of unhelpful behaviour towards patients

Behaviour	Example of source
Overidentification (becoming too close emotionally)	You become overly close to a young patient with a drug addiction problem because your own brother had a similar problem
Underidentification (becoming too distant emotionally)	Due to fatigue and stress, you find it difficult to be warm and empathetic with a patient's distressed relative
Becoming judgemental of patients and their lifestyle	Coming from a family of doctors, you find it difficult to understand why some patients do not comply with their treatment
Becoming didactic in consultations and lecturing a patient	In your own upbringing you were taught to obey people in positions of authority
Always treating the patient's problem without attending to any of the patient's emotional needs	Although you are a good scientist, you find it difficult to respond to a patient's feelings because no one in your own family seemed to attend to anyone else's feelings
Giving the patient unrealistic hope about the likely outcome of his or her illness	You find it difficult talking to a patient about his or her fears and about loss because these are issues that at this time are too close to your own experience, or because you have not seriously thought about them
Feeling under pressure to solve every problem, offer definitive answers to questions and create a feeling of certainty	One reason you were drawn to medicine was your interest in solving problems. In practice, you view it as your duty to rescue people from pain, uncertainty and feelings of loss

Questions to ask yourself about communicating

As a rough guide, the following questions can help you identify the presence and possible source of communication problems in medical practice:

- Take your own 'emotional temperature': are you overly sensitive, or emotionally cold and distant?
- Have you established a pattern that is unhelpful in how you communicate with patients (e.g. are you constantly argumentative or dismissive)?
- Are you frequently tired and irritable (e.g. from too much work, or personal difficulties)?
- Are the boundaries between your personal and professional lives sometimes unclear? Do you take home too much work, or come in to work when it is not necessary to do so?
- Is there a detectable change in your leisure pursuits (e.g. too much drinking and no exercise)?
- Are there significant changes in your family and personal relationships?
- Have you stopped enjoying your work, and do you always look forward to the end of the day?
- Do you feel a sense of achievement in your work (even if you look after very ill patients), or does the constant experience of loss take its toll on you?
- Have colleagues and patients told you that you look tired and stressed?
- Is exam tension interfering with personal and professional relationships?
- Have you started to neglect your own needs and interests?

Hints on self-help

It is important to develop your skills to help manage your workload, professional relationships and some of your feelings. Here are some strategies that may help you to face the challenges you will meet during the course of your training as well as in medical practice.

- Recognise the events that make you stressed, challenged or depressed.
- Recognise the patterns in your behaviour or work schedule that create or exacerbate these stresses.
- Aim to reduce stress by personal and (if necessary) organisational change.
- Re-evaluate your lifestyle and patterns of work in order to prevent a recurrence of overly stressful episodes.
- Aim to improve your experience and skills so that challenges are seen as opportunities, not threats.
- If appropriate, become more assertive.
- Talk to others; discussion with a sympathetic tutor, consultant, hospital chaplain, student counsellor or peer may be beneficial.

Time management

Managing your time effectively will help you to attain your goals and reduce your stress. Time management skills can be learned and we describe some strategies for developing these skills in the section below.

Almost everyone has at some time lamented 'there are just not enough hours in the day' or said to themselves 'why can't I settle down and get on with my work?' Busy professionals struggle with maintaining a healthy work–life balance and also especially with time management. Medical students, and qualified doctors, are certainly no exception. Learning to manage workload and to reduce stress is a vital skill and helps us to focus on achieving goals rather than on being busy.

In order to manage our time, we first have to identify where and how we waste time. For this, we need to understand which situations, tasks or mood states are more likely to lead to avoidance or procrastination. Perhaps we are being distracted by the wrong tasks or putting in too much effort into those which are unimportant. There is a difference between an 'urgent' and an 'important' task. For example, it is *important* to prepare for your examinations, but it is reasonable to assume that it is an *urgent* matter if you have been asked to take a blood sample from a seriously ill patient to the laboratory by the professor of medicine. Furthermore, jumping straight in to manage an urgent task may deflect from the more pressing important one, which simply leaves one feeling stressed.

Assigning priority to tasks is vital and each of us should keep an up-to-date 'to do' list. It does not mean that everything on the list should be done with the same degree of urgency, but by identifying tasks that require our attention and then by assigning priority to them, we are less likely to be overwhelmed, to act impulsively or divert attention to a less pressing problem. It also gives us a sense of achievement to tick them off when they are completed. A 'to do' list should also contain information about the approximate amount of time needed for the given task. This helps us to manage our time and, by rank-ordering the tasks, to avoid becoming stressed by less important tasks.

Procrastination may stem from a fear of failure (or a fear of success!); poor decision-making skills; a poor track record in self-management and organisation; a streak of perfectionism (avoiding tasks unless we can deal with them perfectly); or waiting until 'the time is right' to tackle a pressing task. A first step to overcoming procrastination is to be honest and recognise that you are doing it. You then have to work out why you are procrastinating and work in a very practical and determined way to overcome the problem. For example, if you are avoiding completing some coursework, it may be easier to break the project into manageable proportions and to start on those sections where you can achieve early success and derive satisfaction that can then give you the impetus to continue with the rest.

Set goals for yourself. For example, a personal goal may be to complete the course successfully. You then need to focus on how to achieve this goal. This is where things become practical and even measurable. Think about what you will need in order to achieve your goal. Be specific about the resources that you will need (e.g. time) and whether you will need to change any aspect of your lifestyle in order to achieve your goal. It is always a good idea to write down you goals and the resources needed, framing both positively and precisely. Focus on goals that reflect performance more than outcome. For example, you will focus better on the task if you aim to work hard and to put in extra effort to coursework, rather than setting the goal of being 'top of the class'. Of course, it is important to remember to set realistic goals otherwise you may encounter failure, which will lower your motivation and performance.

Performance can be reduced to a simple formula: behaviour over time. We all have to manage our hopes, goals and expectations within our capabilities and within the time that is available to us. Perhaps you learned at school how to schedule study and revision time. If you did, you will remember that the goal of scheduling was not to cram full every waking moment with studying. It is vital to allocate time for rest, play, socialising and even for the planning and organising of our time!

Assertiveness

Assertiveness is an important component of effective communication. Although some people are naturally more assertive than others, it is possible to develop your assertiveness skills. But what is assertiveness? We all recognise the passive individual who seems to allow others to walk over him or her, and, on the other hand, the aggressive individual who barges in, or automatically assumes command. Between these extremes is the person with appropriate assertiveness skills. It is generally agreed that being assertive enables individuals to:

- act in their own best interests
- express personal rights without denying the rights of others
- stand up for themselves without undue anxiety
- express honest feelings comfortably.

In the majority of situations, assertiveness is appropriate. Moreover, it certainly helps us to cope with the stresses of being a medical student and doctor. We need to remember, though, that, although assertiveness means expressing and supporting one's views, it also involves respecting the views of others. Studies have shown that assertiveness is specific to the situation: in other words, we may be more assertive at work than at home, or vice versa.

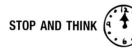

STOP AND THINK

Where would you place yourself on this line?

Non-assertive   *Assertive*   *Aggressive*

←—————————————————————————————————→

What situations might make you move to the right, or to the left?

Features of assertiveness

Non-assertive individuals tend to value themselves below others and show this by being apologetic, avoiding conflict at all cost, often using a soft voice and avoiding eye contact. In contrast, assertive people tend to:

- stand up for themselves but respect the views of others
- not be afraid to express personal feelings and opinions
- in conversation, address the main issues under discussion
- use a firm tone of voice
- demonstrate appropriate body language (i.e. good eye contact, upright posture, etc.).

How to develop assertiveness skills is beyond the scope of this book, but the above points may help you to analyse your own level of assertiveness and give some clues (if you need them) about how to become more assertive.

Relationships with patients

Probably every medical student has at some time been put in the invidious position of being asked by a patient to give information about the patient's medical condition when either they do not know the answer, or feel that they are not yet qualified to provide the information. We may question why patients choose to ask a student when they should ask a nurse or doctor: perhaps they have already been given information but have forgotten it, or perhaps they would like someone else to provide a different view that will give them greater hope.

This can place you in a dilemma: failure to cooperate with the patient's request for information may result in the patient not wanting to help you. The individual could withdraw permission to allow you to clerk and examine him or her. On the other hand, if you do provide information that is either factually incorrect or contradicts the consultant's views and approach to care, you may get yourself into trouble. Always offer to refer the questions to qualified staff, and provide feedback to the staff if you have any concerns.

The role of the student undergoing clinical training is not an easy one, and most qualified staff (and some patients, too) recognise this. Many students feel that it is both self-denigrating and self-defeating to introduce themselves to a patient as a student. After all, what benefit will the patient derive from the contact? Therefore, why should the patient cooperate with the student? Obviously, not every patient will allow students to examine them, but this may reflect the personality of the patient (and degree of illness) rather than your personal attributes or perceived limitations.

It is important not to misrepresent yourself with patients; you are obliged to introduce yourself as a medical student. Make sure that you explain the purpose of your contact with them, what they can expect and how long the procedure or interview is likely to take. Also, explain how your contact with them will benefit your training. Of course, you should offer to assist them in any way you can (e.g. to sit up in bed, to go to the lavatory, etc.). Do not be shy to interrupt the patient once you have started to take a history: some patients may relish the idea of teaching you, and feel that they can best do this by providing an extensive medical history of all that has happened so far. At the end of your contact, remember to thank the patient and explain briefly what has been helpful to you. Not only is this an important courtesy, but it may also make the task easier for the next student who has to clerk the patient.

Relationships with professional colleagues

In this chapter, we have so far addressed some of the important personal issues that influence communication with patients. Many of these are also relevant to communication with professional colleagues and to the teacher–student relationship. Obviously, there is a great difference between the teaching of children at school and the teaching of medical students. Universities encourage independent learning: lectures are designed to introduce new material, while tutorials provide an opportunity to clarify and discuss ideas and skills. Above all, you yourself are expected to read avidly and to fill in the gaps not covered in formal teaching.

Despite the many advances in teaching methods in higher education, several professions – including medicine – continue to rely on the apprenticeship model of learning. In your clinical training and position as a house officer up to registrar grade, you will serve as an apprentice to a more senior and experienced practitioner. The rate at which you learn and your enjoyment of the process depend, to some extent, on the relationship between you and your consultant or teacher. Although the relationship is necessarily hierarchical, the gap appears to narrow as you progress through the stages of training and become socialised into the language and ways of medical practice. Outsiders, incidentally, often remark on the medical jargon that marks a boundary between doctors and laypeople. For an interesting sociological view of this topic, you might care to read the article, 'Medical slang and its functions'.[1]

Written communication about patients

Doctors are trained to communicate with and to other professionals information about their patients using various methods. An essential part of the communication is letter-writing and keeping notes on the physical examination of a patient, as well as on investigations and treatment. The terminology, labels, language and style of written communication about patients all influence the impressions that other professionals form of the patient as well as those of the professional writing. Written communication should always be clear and free from prejudiced views and stereotypical language. In the modern era, we should all be especially careful to avoid sexist, racist, ageist and disablist language in letters and notes, though this is not always easy to achieve, as negative attitudes are deeply embedded in our language. The imbalance of power between patient and doctor should, therefore, be carefully considered when we write about patients: the power to influence patients' lives through written communication should not be underestimated. The fact that patients have access to their medical notes and medical reports written about them (Access to Health Care Records Act 1990[2] and Data Protection Act 1998[3]) means that we must ensure that what we write about patients must not psychologically harm them.

If medical care is to meet its high standard of patient care, patient record keeping should assist by:

- improving continuity between doctor–patient contacts by providing a record of the issues covered with the patient and any findings from investigations or examinations
- facilitating planning and evaluation of progress
- providing data for audit and statistical purposes
- providing a legal record of what happened and when.

Not only should the practice and procedures of record-keeping have a clear purpose, but there should also be clear principles that guide the quality of record-keeping. The NHS training guide to record-keeping, *Just for the Record* (NHS Training Directorate[4]), identifies four principles that underpin patient records, which can be used for auditing patient records. These principles can be classified as:

1. communication
2. legality
3. integration
4. partnership.

The following question may be helpful in deciding what needs to be included in patient notes: 'Does the record clearly communicate the information necessary for other professionals to perform their own care of the patient?'

Good communication is fundamental to good health care and practice. It is helpful to keep in mind the following when thinking about written or verbal communication about patients:

1. One of the purposes of recording information is to ensure care and treatment can be communicated to everyone involved, including the patient. Remember too that patients will soon have access to copies of doctors' letters about them.
2. Poor communication between colleagues is often cited in investigations of patient complaints about doctors.
3. Written records need to present information in a clear, concise and understandable format, keeping in mind the other professionals involved with the patient. Clarity of notes is also particularly important since patients may request access to their records.

With respect to legality, ask yourself whether the patient record could stand up in court or in a professional inquiry. Documentation relating to patient care is a record and all records should conform to standards that safeguard the doctor against unprofessional and unsafe practice. While the main objective of record-keeping is to support the care and treatment process, the growing threat of litigation with which we are all faced in our practice means that we have to remember that notes could be scrutinised in a court of law. It helps to remind yourself when recording notes that you may be asked to justify the standards and clarity of your notes by lawyers, and that in cases of negligence or malpractice they may serve as a defence.

A well-integrated and structured patient record promotes and facilitates an understanding of the progress of health delivery to a patient. All documentation, including letters from patients, reports from professionals and records of telephone calls, should be integrated in one case file. The patient record should progress chronologically and be structured by type of information.

When records are used by more than one professional, the collaboration of professionals in delivering health care to the patient, as well as the patient's needs, should be reflected in the notes. Integrated and structured case records assist the care process and the larger health care system from assessment, to the implementation of treatment, to discharge.

It goes without saying that each patient should have an individual file, the contents of which vary between hospitals and organisations. Records should be kept in a secure and locked location. It is good practice not to move records from the premises where a patient is seen, although this may be unavoidable in cases of home visits. If files do need to be moved from the premises, the following two guidelines may help ensure that confidentiality is maintained:

1. Never leave files in cars or in public view.
2. Have a removable sheet upon which all private biographical details are kept and remove this sheet when records are taken outside the workplace. This will avoid identification of the patient should the file be lost or stolen.

Health trusts often use quality standards to help monitor the levels of practice being achieved and to inform practice changes. The recording of information about patients may be monitored in this way. An example of a basic recording standard may include:

1. All papers should be fastened securely in a file and each sheet identified with the patient's name and date of birth.
2. All entries should be dated and signed.
3. All entries should be written in black ink and be legible.
4. All entries should be chronological and up to date.

Letter-writing

During the first encounter with a patient, ensure that the patient understands that the information considered relevant to a third party may be communicated to that person, subject to the patient's consent. Remember too that patients have the right to be sent copies of all medical correspondence relating to them, and this should guide the style and content of your letters.[5] It is also important to keep in mind to whom the letter is being written. Specialist knowledge by the reader should not be assumed unless the person is already known to the doctor. Specifically, jargon should be avoided. Avoid cluttering the letter or report with lots of detail. Information included should be accurate and specific to the doctor's knowledge or assessment of the patient. It is common practice to start a letter with a courtesy remark, such as: 'Thank you for seeing this patient who…' or 'Thank you for referring…'. Letter-writing is, for most, an acquired art, which is greatly enhanced by reading many examples of letters written by others and developing your own style. We now turn to the challenges of working in teams.

Working in teams

A seasoned doctor once remarked: 'It's not working with patients that causes me stress; it's having to work with colleagues!' These sentiments are echoed by many people across a range of professions. There is something about teamwork, accountability, working within organisations and multidisciplinary teams that adds complexity to our jobs. Some perceive teamwork as a hindrance. Even within 'normal' teams or families, there are disagreements, rivalries, misunderstandings and sometimes escalating tensions, but this does not necessarily destroy the group nor compromise the integrity of the family. These dynamics are frequently encountered within teams and it would a rare team that did not experience internal conflict – or, indeed, external threats – from time to time.

We know that some teams can achieve things that individuals alone could never hope to attain. In health care, this is an accepted fact since problems we encounter are often complex and require the expertise of several or many people. The term *synergy* is used to describe the phenomenon where a group or team can achieve something more than if the individuals were working separately. For example, you could ask 30 people to build a new lecture theatre, but not organise them into a team – in which case, the outcome is likely to be a disaster! No one will know who is responsible for which tasks and there will be no clear understanding of the specific goals and deadlines to be reached. On the other hand, organising the same number of people into a team, clearly describing the overall mission, providing leadership and guidance, monitoring progress, discussing obstacles and delegating tasks is the obvious way to begin construction. Teamwork is core to the practice of health care. It would be frightening to think of surgery being performed on a patient without a clear understanding of the mission, goals, roles and functions of each member of the operating team, and their understanding of who is in charge.

In the 'old' days, doctors were automatically ascribed the role of team leader in health care settings. The rivalry between consultant and matron was legendary, but the authority of the doctor usually went unchallenged. These days, things are different in the health service. This is partly because we have a better understanding of how teams work and we are able to apply scientific methods to organisational processes. There is also an emerging culture of active management, accountability and multidisciplinary teamwork, all of which have made for a more democratic (though, arguably, bureaucratic) approach to team management.

An obvious context for you as a medical student to observe team dynamics is the ward round. It may be helpful to consider the following in relation to teamwork when you next attend a ward round:

1. Are there any clear rules or expectations about relationships in the team that you can identify?
2. Who sits next to whom? What does this convey about relationships?
3. Does the consultant or leader set a positive tone by welcoming everyone, ensuring newcomers are introduced and facilitating discussion? Or is the meeting characterised by fear or apathy?
4. Who speaks and in what order? What does this convey about how the team is organised, either formally or informally?
5. Are everyone's views and opinions solicited, or are only those who speak up or volunteer information heard?
6. What relationship with other professionals (e.g. nurses, physiotherapists, psychologists) is conveyed by how the ward round is conducted? Are their opinions included?
7. How are disagreements managed and resolved?
8. When the ward round is over, is there informal chat between people, or do people rapidly disperse? Where there is informal chat, is this generally light-hearted, or is this the time that people's real feelings are expressed that they were otherwise afraid to display during ward round?
9. How did you feel in your role as medical student? Did you feel included or excluded, welcomed or ignored, respected or patronised?

Picking up from the topic of human error, introduced in Chapter 10, it is now relevant to consider what mediates human performance in teams. A number of factors can be identified, including the work setting, roles and relationships, available skills and how the team is organised. There are some striking examples in aviation, for example, where poor team coordination caused air disasters, and others where the exemplary action of the crew prevented a major catastrophe. Lessons that have been learned from aviation about group behaviour and teamwork have recently been applied to medicine. Although seemingly different from one another, teamwork in medicine and aviation shares a number of common features (Table 12.2):

Table 12.2 Safety in teams: the overlap between medicine and aviation

1. Safety is paramount; bad decisions can prove fatal
2. Staff (or crew) mostly work in teams and individual performance is determined by how teams are managed and organise themselves, as well as the management culture within the organisation
3. Teams usually bring together people with different specialisms and skills; the team must work together effectively even if some of the members have not previously worked together or come from different specialisms
4. Emphasis is placed on communication between members: task-setting, problem-solving, leadership, personality and interpersonal dynamics are all relevant when we think about communication

One obvious difference between aviation and medicine is that pilots are repeatedly tested not only on their own ability to fly (aviate, navigate and communicate), but also on their performance within a team. Although most qualified doctors work within practices or teams, surprisingly few are assessed on their ability to work within or lead a team. This is likely to change in the coming years as greater emphasis comes to be placed on teaching problem-solving skills to medical students and assessing these skills in clinical practice.

Teams generally work effectively and safely when the rules or processes for making decisions are clear to everyone and are adhered to. Good leaders within teams also recognise that all team members should contribute to decision-making but that they are responsible for the final decision. Team leaders can acquire special skills to help them become more effective in their role. These skills may include: eliciting contributions to decision-making, listening skills, using questions to gather information, noting body language and understanding different leadership styles. Of course, as doctors we work in stressful environments, and fatigue, work or personal stress, hunger, emotional arousal and other factors may all affect our judgement, decisions and ability to communicate.

Each team member carries in his or her mind a mental model of how the team works or operates. Each may be different, although not necessarily more accurate than the rest. A good leader should be able to glean from all the available verbal and non-verbal communications how each member perceives the team. The leader should also be willing to try to shift negative or unhelpful ideas where these impede the team's progress. Effective observation and communication skills are, therefore, just as necessary and important for working effectively with our colleagues as they are for doctor–patient consultations.

The medical handover

The practice of exchanging information between health professionals is a neglected topic in the training of doctors, nurses and other health professionals.[6] A handover involves the exchange of clinically relevant information between health professionals about a patient and may take place in a variety of contexts, three of which are highlighted below:

- in a team meeting when, for example, night staff hand over to day staff
- when a patient is transferred to another service or ward
- where important information about duties, tasks and specific directives about treatment and care must be given to another professional or team that assumes responsibility for all or part of a patient's care.

Each context involves: (1) communication between at least two people, either verbally or in written form, including electronically; (2) an exchange of information; (3) a judgement about what is relevant information, and therefore a form of editing; and (4) increased risk to patient safety arising from ambiguity over expectations and directives, incomplete information exchange, misinterpretation of information, as well as certain cognitive and behavioural (known as 'human factors') limitations stemming from fatigue, distraction, work overload and having inadequate time, among others. Sometimes key information is deliberately distorted or withheld in the course of a handover as a means of concealing medical errors or to make a patient's clinical problem seem less complex to another team.

It is important for doctors to learn to communicate with their colleagues about patients effectively, accurately and concisely. With the move toward shift work for junior doctors, the handover assumes greater importance in health care settings and deserves time and effort in order to ensure good and safe practice. It requires:

- Someone to take a lead to ensure that relevant information is exchanged clearly and fully
- An agreed amount of time in which the information can be shared
- A climate in which everyone feels free to ask questions and seek clarification in order to avoid misunderstandings or ambiguity; no one should feel bullied into accepting a situation or information
- Time and space allocated for the task of a handover
- Freedom from distractions (e.g. receiving phone calls or answering pagers)
- Someone to keep written notes about what has been discussed.

Effective learning and teaching

Effective learning and teaching depend on communication skills. Think back to a recent lecture: were students engaged in the learning process? If so, how? Students usually rate the lectures and seminars in which they feel they have been active participants as more successful, as opposed to those in which they are passive auditors subjected to a traditionally didactic teaching session. But students will only actively participate in the learning process if they can expect to receive constructive, positive feedback. Ridicule and criticism from the teacher will hardly endear the student to the teacher or the subject.

A number of negative processes may interfere with how students communicate with teachers and, therefore, how they learn. (These negative processes must be distinguished from the normal feelings of self-doubt and uncertainty that invariably accompany learning.) Unremitting negative feelings associated with learning – and characterised by a deteriorating relationship between student and teacher – should be acknowledged and discussed as a first step towards their resolution. Again, a supportive tutor, hospital chaplain or counsellor can help in this process. The following is a list of the negative feelings that may warrant attention:

- *Feeling deskilled*: Students may have doubts about their abilities resulting from constant questioning of their ideas and practices. They may lack confidence in how they explain ideas (verbally or in coursework), and in their relationships with peers and teachers.
- *Feeling confused*: Encountering new ideas can lead to a period of confusion and uncertainty while the ideas are being assimilated. These feelings can result in a loss of confidence or feelings of frustration.
- *Feeling disconnected from teachers*: Established relationships with teachers may change as you progress through medical school. Supportive relationships may end and new ones start, bringing with them anxiety, uncertainty, hope and expectation. Poor relationships with teachers may be a sign of boredom, personal difficulties or discontent with the course or chosen field of study.
- *Feeling uninterested*: Your personal life may interfere with your ability to concentrate and study. Similarly, some subjects may be dull, or may be taught in an uninteresting way, leading to apathy and boredom.
- *Feeling humiliated and angry*: Sometimes a teacher or consultant will reprimand or criticise a student in front of other students or patients. This can cause upset and lead to a loss of self-confidence.

Handling difficult student–teacher relationships

Because of the hierarchical structure implied in the student–teacher relationship, you may feel unable to speak directly to the teacher concerned, for fear that a discussion may worsen your situation. It is then advisable to talk to a tutor or sympathetic teacher who can possibly reassure you, or be supportive, with the aim of helping to restore your self-confidence. Remember: people who are not good teachers have either not been taught how to teach (perhaps they are recognised for their research and clinical skills), or may themselves have been badly taught – that is, taught in a way that prevented them from asking questions and participating actively in the learning and teaching process.

An experience of bad teaching can help you to think about how you yourself would teach students and junior doctors. There is an isomorphic relationship between teaching skills and communication skills, so you can learn something about how a consultant might communicate with a patient by how the consultant communicates with students. Is the consultant engaging, sympathetic, responsive to your needs and concerns? Does he or she teach at the right pace – not too fast or slow? Does he or she invite questions, feedback and collaboration? Is he or she well prepared, but also sufficiently flexible to deal with unexpected events and problems? There are constant advances in teaching methods in medicine, and you should use these to reflect on your own communication skills with colleagues and patients.

Key points

- Experiences from our own family and upbringing affect how we relate to others and communicate with them.
- We experience different relationships and relate differently as we move through different life stages.
- Rigid patterns of interaction in relationships (e.g. being emotionally too close to patients, or too distant) should be identified and addressed.
- There are emotional processes in learning (and teaching) that influence communication and relationships between students and teachers.
- Medical students are often caught in the middle between the patient and doctor, and may experience role confusion.
- Written communication about patients is an acquired skill, but also has legal consequences; care should be taken to ensure all records are legible, up to date, signed and help others understand what has happened to the patient.
- Communication skills can also help us to understand how people might behave within a team and to navigate around the challenges posed by working within multidisciplinary teams.

FURTHER READING

Groopman J 2007 How doctors think. Houghton Mifflin, Boston

Montgomery K 2005 How doctors think: clinical judgment and the practice of medicine. Oxford University Press, New York

Steinberg D 2000 Letters from the clinic. Routledge, London

REFERENCES

1. Coombs R, Chopra S, Schenk D et al 1993 Medical slang and its functions. Social Science and Medicine 36: 987–989
2. Access to Health Care Records Act 1990 Available online at: www.legislation. hmso.gov.uk
3. Data Protection Act 1998 Available online at: www.legislation.hmso.gov.uk
4. NHS Training Directorate 1995 Just for the record: a guide to record keeping for health care professionals. NHS Training Directorate, Bristol
5. Freedom of Information Act 2000 Copying letters to patients – good practice guidelines. April 2003. Department of Health, London
6. Bernau S, Aldington S, Robinson B et al 2006 From medical student to medical doctor: the medical handover – a good habit to cultivate. Student British Medical Journal 14: 177–220

Exercises

Exercise 1
Open and closed questioning (see pp. 16–17)

This exercise is designed to demonstrate the advantages and disadvantages of using open and closed questions.

1. One member of the group acts as the interviewer and another as the interviewee. The rest of the group are observers.
2. The interviewee chooses a recent personal experience (e.g. a visit to the dentist, a holiday) and tells the interviewer what that experience is.
3. The interviewer must obtain as much information as possible using only closed questions.
4. The observers assess: the time taken; the number of questions; and the information (quality and type) obtained.
5. Now repeat the exercise with other members of the group, but with the interviewer using only open questions.
6. Discuss the advantages and disadvantages of using open and closed questions in an interview.

Exercise 2
Passing on the message (see p. 17)

1. Ask 4–6 members of the group to leave the room.
2. Give the remaining members a copy of this exercise (see telephone message to be passed on, below) and ask them to observe and record how the message is passed on.
3. Ask the first volunteer to come back into the room and give the following instructions.
   - I am going to read you a message once only.
   - Listen carefully and attempt to remember it.

- You must not ask any questions or take any notes.
- You will then have to pass the message on to the next person who comes into the room.
4. After the last volunteer has listened to the message passed on, the observers should report back.
5. Discuss how the volunteers could have been helped to improve their listening.
6. Repeat the exercise using the aids to listening that you have identified.

Telephone message to be passed on

Mr Philips, from Going Far travel agency, phoned about your holiday arrangements. Your flight with Virgin Airlines on Friday 12 July, leaving at 13.20, has been cancelled. The next flight available is with Air India on Monday 15 July at 07.50 hours. You will have to change to Gulf Air in Bahrain, leaving at 16.00, and will arrive in Hong Kong at 05.00 hours on Tuesday 16 July. Please phone Miss Clark on 0208 249 0892 to confirm arrangements before 16.30 today.

7. For each volunteer, tick when the words are repeated correctly. If they are omitted, or repeated incorrectly, leave the square blank.

Details/Students	1	2	3	4	5	6
Mr Philips						
Going Far						
Virgin Airlines						
Friday 12 July						
13.20 hours						
Air India						
Monday 15 July						
07.50 hours						
Gulf Air						
Bahrain						
16.00 hours						
Hong Kong						
05.00 hours						
Tuesday 16 July						
Miss Clark						
0208 249 0892						
Before 16.30 hours						

Exercise 3
Non-verbal listening skills (see p. 19)

1. For this exercise the group breaks into pairs, and the letter A or B is assigned to each member of the pair.
2. Each participant is given one of the written cards below:

Card A (the interviewee)

B will ask you a question. Provide the answer, noting your partner's reaction:

- Is he/she listening?
- Is he/she interested?
- What is it about your partner that helps you assess how attentively he/she is listening to you?
- How does your partner's response make you feel?

Card B (the interviewer)

Ask a simple question (e.g. 'Will you tell me about your journey to work today?') As your partner answers, go to great lengths to appear uninterested. Avoid eye contact, fidget with papers, look at your watch.

---

3. Stop after about 5 minutes.
4. A and B then swap cards and repeat the exercise.
5. Next, another card is given to each A and B in the pairs as follows:

Card A is the same as before.

Card B is different:

Card B2 (the interviewer)

Ask A to tell you something he or she would like to change about him- or herself. Attend carefully to your partner's response. Maintain eye contact and nod at intervals. Make encouraging grunts and noises but no verbal responses.

---

6. Stop after about 5 minutes.
7. Now bring the group together to share and compare their feelings during the exercise.

Exercise 4
Verbal listening skills (see p. 19)

1. As in Exercise 3, the group works in pairs, preferably in different pairs from before. Written cards are again provided.

Card A remains as before:

Card A (the interviewee)

B will ask you a question. Provide the answer, noting your partner's reaction:
- Is he/she listening?
- Is he/she interested?
- What is it about your partner that helps you assess how attentively he/she is listening to you?
- How does your partner's response make you feel?

Card B is different:

Card B3 (the interviewer)

Ask A to tell you about his or her home town.

As your partner answers, interject occasionally, repeating word for word some parts of A's talk. Follow this on by interjecting occasionally – not with their exact words, but summarising the last few words, e.g. 'So what you're saying is . . .'.

---

2. Stop after 5 minutes.
3. A and B then swap cards and repeat the exercise.
4. Next, another card is given to each A and B in the pairs as follows:

Card A is the same as before.

Card B is different:

Card B4 (the interviewer)

Ask A to tell you about an emotionally moving incident from his or her childhood.

Try to reflect your partner's feelings, e.g. 'You feel . . . because . . .' or 'That must make you feel . . .'.

---

5. Again, stop after 5 minutes. A and B swap cards and repeat the exercise. The group is then brought together to share and compare their feelings during the exercise.

[Exercise courtesy of Dr Joe Rosenthal]

Exercise 5
Opening an interview with a patient (see p. 29)

Task 1

1. Arrange yourselves into groups of three or four members (preferably with people you do not know well).
2. Read the case scenario below and then discuss with your group different ways in which you might initiate an interview with the patient.
3. Next, focus on five questions that you think would be useful to start a conversation with the patient in order to: (a) put the patient at ease; and (b) give and elicit information that you think is necessary.
4. When the task is completed, the groups reconvene and discuss their ideas.

Case scenario

Mr Brown is a 42-year-old businessman. The registrar has asked you to check the patient. All you know is that he requires surgical intervention to repair a right inguinal hernia. You do not know what the patient understands about his admission to hospital because you have not yet spoken to him.

Task 2

1. Return to your own group and identify one person to role-play the patient and one person to role-play the medical student. The rest of the group should observe the doctor–patient interaction.
2. All the groups reconvene to give feedback on the exercise (see Appendices A, B and C).

Exercise 6
Breaking bad news (see p. 64)

Learning how to break bad news is difficult. There are few opportunities for live supervision, and role-play exercises may not adequately simulate the real situation. Nonetheless, you can increase your confidence in how to break bad news by practising on a fellow student or friend.

1. Devise a scenario in which bad news must be given. Decide on the nature of the problem and assign roles. Start the role-play and stop after 3 minutes. (Note that most students are good at conveying sympathy and responding to the patient's concerns, but find it difficult to know how to deal with questions that may be unanswerable.)

2. Spend the next 3 minutes of the role-play concentrating on how to deal with 'unanswerable' questions. Your partner should give you constructive feedback and then swap roles.

3. After you have both had a chance to play each role, discuss your individual styles and see what you can learn from one another (as well as about yourself) in handling sensitive and difficult situations (see Appendices A, B and C).

Exercise 7
Taking a sexual history (see p. 80)

Topics for group discussion

1. Think about a medical consultation in which problems relating to sex and reproduction are discussed (e.g. a first assessment of a patient at an infertility clinic; someone needing treatment for a sexually transmitted disease). What issues would you find most embarrassing to talk about with the patient? Can you think of any reasons for your embarrassment? If there is an opportunity, discuss this exercise with a colleague and think about how you can improve your confidence in taking a sexual history.

2. Draw up a list of as many sexual activities as you can think of. What are the terms we use for these activities in clinical settings? Are there 'street language' terms with which you should be familiar? How would you explain any of these activities to a patient if you needed to clarify a term that the patient did not understand?

3. If a 13-year-old girl asked you in clinic for advice about contraception, what issues would you want to discuss with her? How would you go about raising them?

4. How would you counsel someone about the dangers of having unprotected sex with casual partners? If that person was reluctant to use condoms, what could you say that might impress on him or her the risks of unprotected sex?

Exercise 8
Communicating with a family (see p. 128)

1. Bring together a group of students willing to role-play a family (see Appendices A, B and C).

2. The 'family' should devise a problem, and the task of the interviewer is to find out about the problem and how it affects the family. After several minutes, or when the interviewer has gathered sufficient information, the whole group should consider the following:

a. With whom did the interviewer first engage? Why? What effect did it have on others?
b. How did the interviewer gather information?
c. How did the interviewer explore the impact of the problem on family relationships?
d. How did each family member feel: included or excluded? Did each person feel that he or she was given equal time to talk?

3. Each person should be given a chance to interview the family. What are the similarities and differences between interviewing an individual and a family?

Exercise 9
Sharing a secret (see p. 137)

1. Work with a partner. One of you has a secret that you do not want to tell the other. The interviewer should try to get the partner to disclose the secret. Discuss the following: what happens? What helps? What does not help?
2. Now, instead of persuading your partner to disclose the secret, talk about the effect on others of keeping the secret. What happens? What do you learn about resistance in conversation? What happens when you stop trying to persuade someone to see your point of view?
3. Swap roles, and then discuss what you have observed (in the context of medical practice) about secrets between patients, their families and health care professionals.

Exercise 10
Mrs Lazio – a challenging consultation (see p. 162)

This exercise refers to the case example in Chapter 10. Can you think of ways you could have improved the progress made in this consultation? Together with a fellow student, try role-playing a different consultation in which the patient is encouraged to explore her illness and its implications. Try also to increase the rheumatologist's understanding of the patient and her reactions. The crisis happened towards the end of the consultation. Can you think of things the rheumatologist might have said early on in the interview in order to avoid the crisis? Also consider some of the things you might need to know if you had interviewed this patient:

What was Mrs Lazio's understanding of her illness?

1. For most of the consultation, the patient and doctor talked at cross-purposes. How might these misunderstandings affect her health?

2. She had never before taken time off from work. Is this a reflection of how serious (or not) she considered her condition to be?
3. She was obviously concerned that she was getting worse. What ideas did she have about the progression of her illness?
4. How did she rate her illness on a scale with the other problems in her life?

What do we know about her work and personal life?

1. Was she happy working full-time? Was she worried that her job prospects might suffer if she took time off work? (Her husband lost his job for this reason.)
2. Was she otherwise happy with life? Or did she have anxieties about herself or her family?
3. How did her condition affect her personal relationships, or her sex life?
4. Was she depressed? How might we (or she) know?
5. How might a worsening and potentially disabling condition affect her life, or the life she might hope for in the future?
6. Who is Mrs Lazio?

When you have answered these questions, return to Chapter 10 and re-read what happened at the follow-up visit.

Appendix A
Guidelines for using role-plays

Role-playing is an important part of developing good communication skills. Through role-play, the 'doctor' can practise in a relatively safe environment and receive helpful feedback. The 'patient' can learn to understand how individuals are affected in different ways by illness and medical care. Observers serve an important function in role-playing sessions and will find it helpful to use the communication skills checklist in Appendix C whilst watching the role-play. Actors can be used to play the 'patient' and can make an important contribution to the session.

Organising a role-play session

1. Decide what it is you want to achieve in the role-play (e.g. perhaps practise listening skills).
2. You may wish to prepare a script for the 'patient' or, alternatively, to role-play spontaneously a situation which has arisen from the group discussion.
3. Always use the 'patient's' role-name.
4. Make sure that all the participants in the role-play understand what you (as organiser) want them to do.
5. Allocate an agreed amount of time and stick to it.
6. Role-play in a small group. Three is the minimum number – the student doctor, the patient and an observer – each taking a turn at each role.
7. The observer is silent throughout the role-play and takes note of the interaction in general and of the specific skills the student doctor wishes to practise.
8. Give feedback in role-playing: start with the student doctor, then the patient and then the observer (see Appendix B).
9. Finally, you will need to come out of the role-play by asking the student doctor and the patient to say who they are in real life! (This is particularly important when the scenario has proved difficult, or when people have taken on a very different role from their normal life.)

FURTHER READING

Steinert Y 1993 Twelve tips for using role-plays in clinical teaching. Medical Teacher 15: 283–291

Appendix B
Guidelines for giving feedback

Giving and receiving feedback after a role-play session might seem a threatening experience but, if handled correctly, it is a valuable method of learning.

When giving feedback

- Always be positive about each other's performance.
- Identify the good parts of the interview: be specific about what was good and why.
- Finally, discuss the parts that were not so good and what could be modified. When making criticisms, always suggest positive alternatives.

The sequence of the feedback session

1. The interviewer (e.g. the 'doctor') says what he/she thinks he/she did well.
2. The interviewee ('patient') says what was done well.
3. The observer(s) state what he/she thought was done well.
4. The interviewer says what he/she could have done differently to make the interview more effective.
5. The observer(s) comment on those parts of the interview that could have been done differently. It is important to make positive suggestions about how the interview could have been modified.
6. The 'patient' makes positive suggestions about making the interview more effective.
7. The interviewer should be asked how he/she feels about the feedback he/she has received.

Appendix C

Assessment of communication skills

Assessment, with immediate feedback, is an important part of the learning process. It enables the student and teacher to plot the student's progress and to identify strengths and areas that require further work.[1] A communication skills checklist (Table C.1) can be used by observers in role-playing and in video-feedback sessions.

Communication skills are now being assessed in undergraduate and postgraduate examinations. The assessment is usually part of an objective structured clinical examination (OSCE), which consists of a series of stations through which the candidate progresses. Each station examines a particular skill, which may be a practical procedure, e.g. measuring a person's blood pressure as part of a physical examination of the cardiovascular system, or a communication skills station, such as having to break bad news to an actor playing the role of a patient or relative. The candidate is observed by an examiner who completes a checklist. Three examples of stations involving the assessment of a candidate's communication skills are given (see pp. 200–202).

Table C.1 Communication skills checklist

Did the student/doctor:	Yes	No	Comments
Introduce him/herself?			
Use the patient's name?			
Greet the patient?			
Explain his/her role?			
Ensure privacy?			
Ensure the patient was comfortable?			
Establish eye contact?			
Use eye contact?			
Allow the patient to complete his/her initial statement?			
Use mainly open questions?			
If the 'doctor' took notes, did he/she inform the patient that he/she would do so?			
If the 'doctor' took notes, was he/she able to do so and still demonstrate interest in the patient?			
Identify and respond to patient's verbal cues?			
Identify and respond to patient's non-verbal cues?			
Provide a summary of what the patient has told him/her?			
Let the patient have the last word?			
Give a pleasant thank you and goodbye?			

Objective structured clinical examination (OSCE)

Station 1: Headache history

Instructions for the candidate: Jane Foster has been referred by her GP to a general medical clinic with a history of headache. You are a medical student. Please explore the presenting complaint in detail, including areas of questioning relevant to it. Do not do a system review.

You have 5 minutes for this station.

Examiner's checklist

Items:

		2	1	0
1.	General approach to patient – introduces self, establishes rapport, eye contact, not patronising/arrogant, courteous	☐	☐	☐
2.	Begins with open questions and moves to closed questioning. Interrupts appropriately, but not interrogative in style	☐	☐	☐
3.	Asks questions about original presentation to GP	☐	☐	☐
4.	Enquires about specific features of headache (character, site, radiation)	☐	☐	☐
5.	Asks questions about timing of headache in relation to onset and whether it varies during the day and night	☐	☐	☐
6.	Asks about precipitating and relieving factors, including posture and coughing, etc.	☐	☐	☐
7.	Enquires about factors that ease and relieve the headache	☐	☐	☐
8.	Asks about associated symptoms	☐	☐	☐
9.	Enquires about any relevant past medical history and family history	☐	☐	☐
10.	Responds appropriately to patient's concerns and views	☐	☐	☐
11.	Listens attentively to what the patient says	☐	☐	☐

2 = Done appropriately and completely
1 = Done to some extent
0 = Not done/not done appropriately

Objective structured clinical examination (OSCE)

Station 2: Communication skills: breast lump

Instructions for the candidate: this patient has recently had an excision biopsy on a lump in her breast and has come to get the results of the biopsy. Explain the biopsy results to the patient.

You have 5 minutes for this station.

Examiner's checklist

Items:	2	1	0
1. Appropriate information – introduces self, establishes rapport, explains role	☐	☐	☐
2. Establishes what the patient understands and expects from the consultation before starting explanation	☐	☐	☐
3. Gives an outline of what he/she is going to cover in the consultation	☐	☐	☐
4. Encourages the patient to ask questions throughout the consultation	☐	☐	☐
5. Gives information at a pace the patient can digest, in small chunks	☐	☐	☐
6. Tells the patient that the biopsy shows that the lump is benign	☐	☐	☐
7. Gives explanation in lay language first before giving medical terms	☐	☐	☐
8. Checks throughout that patient understands, by picking up non-verbal cues or asking directly	☐	☐	☐
9. Asks patient if she has any concerns and identifies her perspective on the situation	☐	☐	☐
10. Responds appropriately when asked for information he/she does not have immediately to hand	☐	☐	☐
11. Summarises at the end of the interview and agrees an immediate plan	☐	☐	☐
12. Provides honest and accurate information to the patient	☐	☐	☐
13. Provides comprehensive information to the patient	☐	☐	☐
14. Provides easily understandable information to the patient	☐	☐	☐
15. Demonstrates empathy with the patient's anxiety	☐	☐	☐
16. Provides appropriate reassurance	☐	☐	☐

2 = Done appropriately and completely
1 = Done to some extent
0 = Not done/not done appropriately

Objective structured clinical examination (OSCE)

Station 3: Communication skills

Instructions for the candidate: this patient was admitted yesterday with an acute asthma attack. Take a history of the presenting complaint, relevant social history and explore the patient's views of his/her problem. You have 5 minutes for this station.

Examiner's checklist

Items:	2	1	0
1. Greeting – says 'hello', 'good morning', uses patient's name, etc.	☐	☐	☐
2. Introduction – states own name and status and purpose of interview	☐	☐	☐
3. Appropriate eye contact (comfortable level) and open posture to indicate attentive listening	☐	☐	☐
4. Facilitation of patient history – nods head, 'mm-hmm', repeats patient's last statement, etc.	☐	☐	☐
5. Appropriate pace and flow – allows patient time to process thoughts and feelings, interrupts appropriately to redirect if patient strays	☐	☐	☐
6. Appropriate mix of questions (open, focused and closed), refrains from interrogative questioning	☐	☐	☐
7. Clear questions and avoidance of jargon, technical or ambiguous wording	☐	☐	☐
8. Explores patient's views on the problem	☐	☐	☐
9. Uses empathy	☐	☐	☐
10. Summarises – checks with patient what has been understood for accuracy and completeness	☐	☐	☐
11. Closes by thanking patient	☐	☐	☐

2 = Done appropriately and completely
1 = Done to some extent
0 = Not done/not done appropriately

REFERENCE
1. Makoul G, Schofield T 1999 Communication teaching and assessment in medical education: an international consensus statement. Patient Education and Counselling 137: 191–195

Appendix D

Presentation: hints and assessment

Key hints for giving a presentation

1. Good preparation is essential

- Prepare your talk carefully.
- Write notes you can refer to easily during your talk.
- Practise – to yourself or to others, and time yourself.
- Ensure that your presentation will not overrun the allotted time.

2. The presentation

Beginning

- Look at your audience and speak clearly.
- Outline what you are going to say – 'the headlines'.

Middle

- Go through the main points one by one.
- Do not read out your notes/overheads – talk to the audience.
- Don't overload the audience with facts/ideas.
- Remember the material is familiar to you but may not be to them.

End

- Summarise the main points.
- Ask for questions.

3. Using the overhead projector

- One or two points/ideas per transparency – do not overload it.
- Use large, clear lettering – typescript if possible.
- Make sure the transparency is in the right position on the screen.

● Address the audience, not the screen.
● Stand clear of the projected image.

4. Using PowerPoint

● Most of the above tips apply to using PowerPoint for your presentations.
● Remember to use a clear font and avoid fussy backgrounds.
● *Always* try to practise with the equipment you will be using.
● Have a back-up (e.g. overheads) in case the equipment fails.

Assessment of small group presentations

Many exercises involve group work and presentations. You could set up one or more of these sessions to get the group to practise formally assessing a presentation and giving feedback.

Criteria for assessment

Preparation: Done background work, knows what he/she is talking about

Clarity: Of speech and materials used (overheads/handouts) and understandable, not overloaded with facts

Structured: Beginning/middle/end, clear objectives, good summary, clear signposting of different stages

Pace: Well paced (not too fast/slow, finish on time)

Interesting: Uses different media (e.g. flipchart, overhead projector, talking, questions), change presenters (when appropriate)

Interactive: Talks to the audience/eye contact, involves audience (e.g. using questions), tone of voice (interested/ enthusiastic)

Date:

Title:

Group members:

What went well?

What could he/she do better?

> Grading system
> 1 = poor; 2 = fair; 3 = average; 4 = good; 5 = excellent
>
> Overall grade out of 5:

Further reading

During the preparation of this book, we found the following publications particularly helpful, in addition to those listed at the end of each chapter. We include them here partly to help students who want to delve deeper into the issues discussed, and also for those involved in helping students to develop their communication skills.

Aspergren K 1999 Teaching and learning communication skills in medicine: a review with quality grading of articles. Medical Teacher 21: 563–570

Ayers S, Baum A, McManus C et al (eds) 2007 Psychology, health and medicine. Cambridge University Press, Cambridge (there are a number of useful articles in this multiauthor book)

Bor R, Gill S, Miller R et al 2008 Counselling in health care settings. Palgrave Macmillan, Basingstoke

British Medical Association 2003–2004 Communication skills education for doctors. BMA, London

Cole SA, Bird J 2000 The medical interview: the three function approach. Mosby, Missouri

Groopman J 2007 How doctors think. Houghton Mifflin, Boston

Hall A, Kidd J 2007 Teaching communication skills. In: Ayers S, Baum A, McManus C et al (eds) Psychology, health and medicine. Cambridge University Press, Cambridge (a concise summary of the teaching and assessment of communication skills)

Hope T, Savulescu J, Hendrick J 2003 Medical ethics and law. Churchill Livingstone, Edinburgh (an excellent introduction covering the core curriculum of ethics and law: well referenced)

Kurtz S, Silverman J, Draper J 2005 Teaching and learning communication skills in medicine, 2nd edn. Radcliffe Medical Publishing, Oxford (intended to be used by both teachers and learners but with emphasis on the teaching of communication skills)

Maguire P, Pitceathly C 2002 Key communication skills and how to acquire them. British Medical Journal 325: 697–700

McManus C, Vincent CA, Thom S et al 1993 Teaching communication skills to clinical students. British Medical Journal 306: 1322–1327

Montgomery K 2005 How doctors think: clinical judgment and the practice of medicine. Oxford University Press, New York

Neighbour R 1987 The inner consultation. MTP, Lancaster (a stimulating guide to 'developing an effective and intuitive consulting style')

Schon D A 1987 Educating the reflective practitioner. Jossey-Bass, San Francisco

Silverman J, Kurtz S, Draper J 2005 Skills for communicating with patients, 2nd edn. Radcliffe Medical Publishing, Oxford (an excellent comprehensive text)

Simpson M, Buckman R, Stewart M et al 1991 Doctor–patient communication: the Toronto consensus statement. British Medical Journal 303: 1385–1387

Stewart MA, Brown JB, Weston WW et al 2003 Patient-centred medicine: transforming the clinical method. Radcliffe Medical Publishing, Oxford

Tuckett D, Boulton M, Olson C et al 1985 Meetings between experts: an approach to sharing ideas in medical consultations. Tavistock Publications, London

Websites

www.bma.org.uk: the British Medical Association website is particularly good for its guidance on ethical issues such as consent and confidentiality

www.dh.gov.uk/consent: this is the website of the Department of Health. Their guide on consent is available here

www.gmc-uk.org/guidance: all publications of the General Medical Council can be accessed, including *Good Medical Practice*

www.legislation.hmso.gov.uk: this website includes all UK statutes from 1987, including those mentioned in this book, i.e. the Data Protection Act 1998, Access to Health Care Records Act 1990 and Mental Capacity Act 2005

www.pickereurope.org: the Picker Institute works to promote understanding of the patient's perspective at all levels of health care policy and practice. Their website gives access to their papers and reports

Subject Index

Page numbers in italics *refer to tables or figures.*

A

Access the Health Care Records Act
    (1990), 179
active listening, 18, 19
    breaking bad news, 69–70
adequacy, information giving, 50
adolescents, 111–125, *117–119*
    help seeking, 123
adverse events, 140–141
age
    sexual history taking, 77
    speech and/or hearing problems,
        154
    see also adolescents, children
aggressive patients, 151–152, *152*
aide-mémoires, medical history
    taking, 45
anger, 151–152, *152*
    breaking bad news, 73
anxiety, 49, 150–151, *151*
    communication effects, 10, 11
    information receiving, 51
appearance
    communication with children, 114
    medical interview, 37
    uncommunicative patients, 148
appropriate behaviour, 149–152
appropriate language, information
    giving, 52–53
assertiveness, 176–177
assumptions
    cultural background, 90
    sexual history taking, 78
    uncommunicative patients, 157

B

authority, informed patients, 166
avoidance, uncommunicative
    patients, 156

bad news *see* breaking bad news
barriers, cultural background, *94,*
    94–96
basic information, medical histories,
    30
beginning of medical interviews, 13,
    29
behaviour
    appropriate, 149–152
    medical interview, 37
    uncommunicative patients, 148
Bengali, 95
    personal names, 91
bias, interpreters, 103
body system review, medical
    interviews, 35–38, *36*
breaking bad news, 60–79, *65*
    case examples, 71–72
    children, 120–121, *121*
    colleagues, examples from, 62
    colleagues, handover to, 71
    complex information, 66
    concerns, 69–70
    coping with, 70
    definition, 60–61
    denial, 68
    difficulties, 61–63, *62*
    empathy, 67
    exercises, 64–65, 191–192

feedback, 69–70, 71
follow-up, 71
giver, 63
hope, 64
infant abnormalities, 74–75
infectious diseases, 64
information giving, 69–70, 120,
    121
life transitions, 62
listening, 67
objective structured clinical
    examination (OCSE), 201
patient knowledge, 67–69
patient reactions, 62, 72–74, *73*
personal loss, 62
personal preparation, 65
physical positioning, 66
physical setting, 65–66
privacy, 66
props, 66
reassurance, 64
recipients, 63
referral, 71
responding to concerns, 66–70
sense of control, 68–69
suicide threats, 73–74
timing, 64
treatment information, 70
violence, 73
burial practices, Judaism, 102

C

Cambridge–Calgary medical
    interview guides, 43–45, *44*

cardiovascular system, medical
      interview, 37
card system, cultural problems, 96
care perception, cultural
      background, 95–96, *100*
carers, uncommunicative patients,
      159
case examples
   adolescents, 117–119
   beginning an interview, 13, 29
   breaking bad news, 71–72
   chronic illness, 104–105,
      117–119
   closed questions, 15–16
   cues, 18
   cultural background, 90, 104–109
   doctor-centred consultations, 24
   HIV infection, 85–86
   impotence, 86–87
   mistakes, 141–142, 142–143
   open questions, 15–16
   patient-centred consultations, 24
   secrecy, 136–137
   sexual history taking, 85–87
   smoking cessation, 55
   uncommunicative patients,
      159–165
children, 111–125, *112*
   breaking bad news, 120–121, *121*
   chronic illness, 119–120
   confidentiality, 124
   consulting room, 114
   direct addressing, 115–116
   doctors' appearance, 114
   drawings, 112–113
   feelings assessment, 116
   gathering information, 114–115
   introductions, 114
   isolation issues, 119–120
   levels of communication, *122*
   parental input, 115, 116
   parental liaison, 121, *122*, 123
   parental overnight stays, 133
   physical environment, 113–114
   play, 112–113
   play areas, 113
   play materials, 113
   professional colleagues, 124
   separation issues, 119–120
   teachers, 124
   toys, 112–113
   understanding, 112
   verbal interaction, 111–112
Chinese families, 95
chronic illness
   case examples, 104–105, 117–119

children, 119–120
   communicating with children,
      116
clarification, 20
closed questions, 15–16
   exercises, 187
cognitive function, medical
      interview, 38
collaboration, informed patients, 168
colleagues
   cultural background consultation,
      103
   handover to, 71
   relationships with, 178
colloquialisms, sexual history
      taking, 84
comfort, interaction with children,
      115–116
communal identity, culture, 94
communication skills, 9–27
   assessment of, 198–202
   development of, 6
   indicators, 171–176
   objective structured clinical
      examination (OCSE), 202
   poor *see* poor communication
   self-help, 174
   self-questioning, 173–174
   training, 4–6
competency, informed consent, 58
complaints, 143–145
   dealing with, 144, *144*
   poor communication, 143–144
   prevention, 145
complex information, breaking bad
      news, 66
complex questions, 16–17
compliance
      see treatment compliance
compliments, communicating with
      children, 116
comprehensivity, sexual history
      taking, 82–83
concentration, information
      receiving, 50
concerns
   breaking bad news, 66–70, 69–70
   family communication, 133–134
   medical interviews, 46–48
   responding to, 66–70
confidentiality
   children, 124
   Hippocratic oath, 135
   interpreters, 157–158
   medical interviews, 47
   patient records, 180

secrecy, 137
congratulation, communicating
      with children, 116
consultations, patient-centred,
      23–25
consulting rooms, communicating
      with children, 114
context, in communication, 172
conversational questions, 17
coping, breaking bad news, 70
counselling, infant abnormality
      information, 75
couples, working with, 132–133
crying
   breaking bad news, 73
   medical interviews, 47–48
cues, 18–19
cultural background, 89–110
   assumptions, 90
   barriers due to, *94*, 94–96
   card system, 96
   care perception, 95–96, *100*
   case examples, 90, 104–109
   colleague consultation, 103
   communal identity, 94
   definition, 90
   discussion of, 97–109
   doctors' background, 96–97
   dress, 92
   family members, 95
   food and diet, 91–92
   gender differences, 105–106
   HIV infection, 96
   human development, 95
   hygiene and grooming, 92
   illness perception, 95–96, 100,
      100
   importance, 89
   indirect questioning, 98–99
   individual identity, 94
   interpreters, 102–103
   introductions, 98–99
   issue responsibility, 92–93
   language, 96
   names/naming, 91, 98
   perceptions, 95–96
   psychological information, 99
   relative consultations, 101–103,
      102
   religions, 92
   setting, 97–98
   sexual history taking, 78
   significant others, 91
   social networks, 103
   treatment balance, 101
   treatment perception, 95–96, *100*

D

Data Protection Act (1998), 43, 179
dealing with complaints, 144, *144*
death practices, Hindus, 102
definition (of communication), 1,
    2, 3
dementia, 158
denial
    breaking bad news, 68
    infant abnormality information,
        75
    information giving, 134
    uncommunicative patients, 154
depression, 149
developing awareness,
        uncommunicative patients,
        153
development of communication
        skills, 6
diagnosis
    communication role, 3
    investigations, *30*
    medical history, *30*
    from patient, 31
    physical examination, *30*
diet, cultural background, 91–92
direct addressing, children, 115–116
disclosure, Hippocratic oath, 135
discomfort, physical examination,
        22
distance between people, 11
doctor-related factors, *10*, 10–11
doctors' cultural background, 96–97
drawings
    children, 112–113
    infant abnormality information,
        74
    information giving, 53
dress, cultural background, 92
drinking history, 41–42
drug history, 42

E

effective listening, 18
efficacy, communication skills
        training, 5
embarrassment, sexual history
        taking, 77
emotional patients, medical
        interviews, 47–48
empathy, 22–23
    anxiety, 150–151
    breaking bad news, 67
encouragement, communicating
        with children, 116
ending of medical interviews, 21

environment *see* physical
        environment/setting
exercises
    breaking bad news, 64–65,
        191–192
    closed questions, 187
    family communication, 192–193
    listening, 17–18
    medical interviews, 191
    messages, 17–18, 187–188
    non-verbal cues, 189
    open questions, 187
    secrecy, 193
    sexual history taking, 192
    uncommunicative patients,
        193–194
    verbal listening skills, 190
existing knowledge, information
        receiving, 50
expectations of patient, 28
extreme reactions, breaking bad
        news, 62
eye contact, 19

F

facial expressions, 19
facilitation, 19
familiarity, cultural background, 89
family communication, 126–138,
        127
    concerns and fears, 133–134
    exercises, 192–193
    guidelines, 134–135
    HIV infection, 129
    identification of family, 128–129
    influence on care, 130–131
    secrecy, 135
    treatment compliance, 131–132
    uncommunicative patients, 159
family history, medical interviews,
        39–40
family members
    cultural issues, 95
    information giving, 134
family names, 98
family support, 127
    observation of, 128
family therapists, 123
family trees, 128–129, *129*
    medical, 40, *40*
fears, family communication,
        133–134
feedback, 197
    breaking bad news, 69–70, 71
    training in, 5–6
feelings assessment, children, 116
follow-up, breaking bad news, 71

food, cultural background, 91–92
forms, informed consent, 57

G

gender differences
    cultural background, 105–106
    sexual history taking, 78
general practice
    consulting room effects, 11
    medical history taking, 43
genetically determined diseases,
        39–40
genitourinary system, medical
        interview, 37
gestures, 19
goal setting, time management,
        175–176
Good Medical Practice, 26–27
grooming, cultural background, 92

H

handover to colleagues, 71
headache history, objective
        structured clinical
        examination (OCSE), 200
health education, sexual history
        taking, 84
hearing problems,
        uncommunicative patients,
        153–156, *155*
hepatitis C, 80
hereditary diseases, 39–40
Hindus
    death practices, 102
    personal names, 91, 98
Hippocratic oath, 25
    disclosure, 135
histories *see* medical histories
HIV infection, 80
    case examples, 85–86
    culture, 96
    family effects, 129
hope, breaking bad news, 64
human development, cultural
        background, 95
hygiene, cultural background, 92

I

identification, patient notes, 42
illness perception, cultural
        background, 95–96, 100, *100*
importance (of communication),
        3–4
impotence, case examples, 86–87
indicators, communication skills,
        171–176

indirect questioning, 98–99
individual identity, culture, 94
individual secrets, 135
infant abnormalities, breaking bad
    news, 74–75
infant deaths, 75
infectious diseases, breaking bad
    news, 64
information gathering, children,
    114–115
information giving, 49–59
    adequacy, 50
    appropriate language, 52–53
    breaking bad news, 69–70, 120, *121*
    denial, 134
    description of, 51–52
    drawings, 53
    family members, 134
    guidelines, *51*
    importance, 53
    lifestyle advice, 56
    management negotiation, 53–54
    patient understanding, 52, 54
    patient views, 53
    person receiving, 50–51
    problem understanding, 52
    written information, 56–57
information receiving
    existing knowledge, 50
    patient cooperation, 51
    understanding, 51
information relevance, 20
information technology, informed
    patients, 165–166
informed consent, 57–59
    forms, 57
    understanding, 57
    voluntariness, 58
informed patients, 165–168
    authority, 166
    collaboration, 168
    control, 166
    information technology, 165–166
internal secrets, 135
interpreters
    bias, 103
    confidentiality, 157–158
    cultural background, 102–103
    uncommunicative patients,
        157–158
interviews *see* medical interviews
introductions
    children, 114
    cultural background, 98–99
    sexual history taking, 82
investigations, diagnosis, *30*
isolation issues, children, 119–120

J

Japanese families, 95
Judaism burial practices, 102
judgmental attitudes, *173*
Just for the Record (NHS Training
    Development), 179

L

language
    appropriate, 52–53
    cultural background, 96
leading questions, 16–17
learning (of communication), 4–6,
    184–186
legality, patient records, 179–180
letter-writing, 180–181
lifelong learning, 7
lifestyle advice, 54–56
    information giving, 56
    negotiation, 56
    patient attitudes, 55–56
    patient support, 56
    seriousness, 55
    solutions, 56
    susceptibility, 55
lifestyle, social history, 41–42
life transitions, breaking bad news,
    62
listening, 17–19
    active *see* active listening
    breaking bad news, 67
    effective, 18
    exercises, 17–18
litigation, 145
location, presenting problems, 33

M

management *see under* treatment
medical family trees, 40, *40*
medical handovers, 183–184
medical histories, 29–42, *30*
    basic information, 30
    diagnosis, *30*
    past, 38–39
    practical hints, 45
    presenting problems
        see presenting problems
    sequence modification, 43
        see also medical interviews
medical interviews, 11–15, 28–48
    beginning of, 13, 29
    body system review, 35–38, *36*
    Cambridge–Calgary guides,
        43–45, *44*
    concerns, 46–48

    ending of, 21
    exercises, 191
    family history, 39–40
    guidelines, *14*
    main part, 14
    opening, 191
    settings, 11
    social history, 40–42
        see also medical histories
medical problems, sexual problems,
    79
mental state review, 37
message taking, exercises, 17–18,
    187–188
misconceptions, sexual history
    taking, *78*
mistakes, 139–143
    case examples, 141–142, 142–143
    causes, 141
    consequences, 143
    recording of, 143
    response to, 142–143
modesty, physical examination, 22
modifying factors, presenting
    problems, 34
mood, medical interview, 37–38
'more-of-the-same' situation,
    treatment compliance, *131*,
    131–132
Muslims, 101
    food and diet, 91
    naming, 98

N

names/naming
    cultural background, 91, 98
    personal *see* personal names
negotiation, lifestyle advice, 56
non-judgemental approach, sexual
    history taking, 83–84
non-verbal cues, 19
    exercises, 189
    medical interview, 37
notes, medical history taking, 45

O

objective structured clinical
    examination (OCSE),
    200–202
    breaking bad news, 201
    communication skills, 202
    headache history, 200
occupational history, 41
occurrence timing, presenting
    problems, 34
opening of medical interviews, 191

open questions, 15–16
  exercises, 187
outpatient clinics
  communication effects, 11
  medical history taking, 43
overidentification, *173*

P

parents
  input, 115, 116
  liaison, 121, *122*, 123
  overnight stays, 133
past medical histories, 38–39
patient(s)
  access to notes, 42, 178–179
  breaking bad news, 72–74
  communication role in
    satisfaction, 3, 49
  cooperation in information
    receiving, 51
  diagnosis from, 31
  expectations, 28
  information giving, 53
  informed *see* informed patients
  knowledge in breaking bad news,
    67–69
  lifestyle advice, 56
  lifestyle attitudes, 55–56
  questions from, 47
  refusal of medical interviews, 46
  relationships with, 177–178
  social history, 41
patient-centred consultations, 23–25
patient notes, 42–43
  patient access, 178–179
patient records, 179–180
  confidentiality, 180
  multi-use, 180
patient-related factors, communication
    effects, 9–10, *10*
patient understanding
  information giving, 52, 54
  presenting problems, 35
  uncommunicative patients, 158
personal attitudes, sexual history
    taking, 78, 81
personal development, 171, *172*
personal issues, 170–186
personality, uncommunicative
    patients, 148
personal loss, breaking bad news, 62
personal names
  Bengali, 91
  Hindus, 91, 98
  Muslims, 98
personal preparation, breaking bad
    news, 65

personal safety, sexual history
    taking, 81
person receiving, information
    giving, 50–51
physical attacks, 151
physical environment/setting
  breaking bad news, 65–66
  children, 113–114
  cultural background, 97–98
  medical interviews, 11
  presenting problems, 34
  sexual history taking, 80–81
physical examinations
  communication during, 22
  diagnosis, *30*
  discomfort, 22
physical positioning, breaking bad
    news, 66
play areas, children, 113
play, children, 112–113
play materials, children, 113
poor communication
  complaints, 143–144
  results of, 4
posture, 19
preoccupation, communication
    effects, 11
presentations, 203–204
presenting problems, 31–35
  history of, *32*, 32–35
  sexual history taking, 82
  sexual problems, 78–79
prevention, complaints, 145
priority assessment, time
    management, 175
privacy
  breaking bad news, 66
  communication effects, 11
probing questions, 16
problems, 147–169
procrastination, time
    management, 175
professional colleagues, children, 124
professionalism, 25–27, *26*
props, breaking bad news, 66
psychological information, cultural
    background, 99
purposeful discussions, sexual
    history taking, 82
purposes (of communication), *3*

Q

quality of life, presenting
    problems, 35
quality, presenting problems, 33
questions, 14–17
  to be avoided, 16–17

closed *see* closed questions
complex, 16–17
conversational, 17
forgetting of, 47
indirect, 98–99
leading, 16–17
open *see* open questions
from patient, 47
simple, 17
subtle, 17

R

radiation, presenting problems, 33
Ramadan, 101
rapport, interaction with
    children, 115
reassurance, breaking bad news, 64
recipients, breaking bad news, 63
records, mistakes, 143
referral, breaking bad news, 71
reflection, 20
relative consultations, cultural
    background, 101–103, *102*
relevant information, 20
religions, cultural background, 92
respiratory system, medical
    interview, 37
role playing, 195–196
routine, childhood chronic illness,
    119–120

S

safety alarms, 152
satisfaction of patient, 3
seating arrangements,
    communication
    effects, 11, *12*
secrets/secrecy, 135–136, *136*
  case examples, 136–137
  confidentiality, 137
  exercises, 193
  family communication, 135
  individual, 135
  internal, 135
self-help, communication skills, 174
self-questioning, communication
    skills, 173–174
seniority, infant abnormality
    information, 74
sense of control
  breaking bad news, 68–69
  informed patients, 166
separation issues, children, 119–120
seriousness, lifestyle advice, 55
setting *see* physical environment/
    setting

severity, presenting problems, 33–34
sexual dysfunctions, 77
sexual harassment, 79
sexual history taking, 77–88
    case examples, 85–87
    comprehensivity, 82–83
    culture, 78
    decision algorithm, 81
    embarrassment, 77
    exercises, 192
    gender differences, 78
    guidelines, 80–88
    health education, 84
    importance, 77–78
    introductions, 82
    misconceptions, 78
    non-judgemental approach, 83–84
    personal attitudes, 78, 81
    personal safety, 81
    presenting problems, 82
    purposeful discussions, 82
    setting, 80–81
    specialists, 84
    stereotypes, 78
    "street language,", 84
    terminology, 84
    timing, 78–79
    who from, 79–80
sexually transmitted infections, 77
sexual problems, 78–79
shared secrets, 135
significant others, cultural background, 91
signposting, 20–21
signs and symptoms, presenting problems, 34
signs of distress, uncommunicative patients, 153
silence, 20
simple questions, 17
smoking cessation, 54
    case examples, 55
smoking history, 41
social development, 172
social distances, uncommunicative patients, 154
social history, medical interviews, 40–42
social networks, cultural background, 103
social problems, sexual problems, 79
social support, 127
solutions, lifestyle advice, 56
specialists, sexual history taking, 84

special problems, 147–169
speech, medical interview, 37
speech problems, 153–156, 155
state of mind, uncommunicative patients, 148
stereotypes, sexual history taking, 78
"street language," sexual history taking, 84
stress, 49
    social history, 42
subtle questions, 17
suicide threats, breaking bad news, 73–74
summarizing, 21
susceptibility, lifestyle advice, 55

T

teachers, communicating with children, 124
teaching (of communication), 184–186
team dynamics, 182, 182–183
team working, 181–183
terminology, sexual history taking, 84
thought content, medical interview, 38
time management, 174–176
    goal setting, 175–176
    priority assessment, 175
    procrastination, 175
time, medical history taking, 45
timing
    breaking bad news, 64
    infant abnormality information, 74
    presenting problems, 33
    sexual history taking, 78–79
tiredness, communication effects, 11
touch, 21–22
toys, communicating with children, 112–113
treatment
    breaking bad news, 70
    cultural perceptions, 95–96
    negotiation of, 53–54
    plans, 28, 28
    results, communication role, 4, 49
treatment balance, cultural background, 101
treatment compliance
    communication role, 49
    family communication, 131–132
    'more-of-the-same' situation, 131, 131–132
treatment perception, cultural background, 100

U

uncommunicative patients, 147–165, 150, 156
    appearance, 148
    assumptions, 157
    avoidance, 156
    behaviour, 148
    case examples, 159–165
    dementia, 158
    denial, 154
    developing awareness, 153
    do not ignore, 156
    exercises, 193–194
    experiences, 148
    family and carer help, 159
    forms of communication, 157
    interpreters, 157–158
    patient understanding, 158
    personality, 148
    signs of distress, 153
    social distances, 154
    speech and/or hearing problems, 153–156, 155
    state of mind, 148
    unconsciousness, 158–159
unconsciousness, uncommunicative patients, 158–159
underidentification, 173
understanding
    anxiety, 151
    children, 112
    information receiving, 51
    informed consent, 57
unhelpful behaviour, 173

V

verbal abuse, 151
verbal cues, 18
verbal interaction, children, 111–112
verbal listening skills, exercises, 190
violence, breaking bad news, 73
visiting hours, 91
visitor restrictions, 91
vocal characteristics, 19
voluntariness, informed consent, 58

W

ward rounds, 45–46, 46
wards, communication effects, 11
written information
    about patients, 178–180
    information giving, 56–57